THE TRUTH ABOUT GARDEN REMEDIES

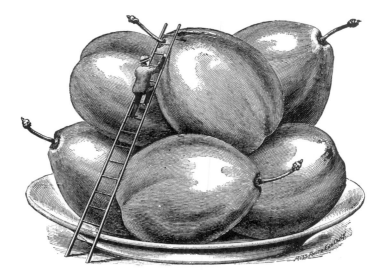

THE TRUTH
ABOUT
GARDEN
REMEDIES

What Works,
What Doesn't
& Why

Jeff Gillman

TIMBER PRESS

Published in 2006 by
Timber Press, Inc.
The Haseltine Building
133 S.W. Second Avenue, Suite 450
Portland, Oregon 97204-3527, U.S.A.
www.timberpress.com

For contact information regarding editorial, marketing, sales, and distribution in the United Kingdom, see www.timberpress.co.uk.

Printed in China

Library of Congress Cataloging-in-Publication Data
Gillman, Jeff, 1969–
    The truth about garden remedies : what works, what doesn't, and why / Jeff Gillman.
        p. cm.
    Includes bibliographical references and index.
    ISBN-13: 978-0-88192-748-1
    ISBN-10: 0-88192-748-1
    1. Garden pests—Biological control. 2. Plant diseases. 3. Plants, Protection of. 4. Organic gardening. I. Title.
    SB975.G55 2006
    632'.96—dc22
                                                        2005015647
A catalog record for this book is also available from the British Library.

To my girls
Suzanne and Catherine
and to
Hy and Ellen Gillman,
who got me started in life, and
Dan Horton,
who got me started
in horticulture

Contents

Preface

EVERYONE seems to have a product, a suggestion, or a little-known secret for making your garden the envy of the neighborhood. Sometimes these amazing tidbits are in a book of household remedies, sometimes they are incorporated into a new product, and sometimes they are offered as an old, forgotten pearl of wisdom in a local newspaper or on a Web site. But how are we to know if these miracle products and plant cures work? Are we just supposed to take someone's word for it? Is there some way to find out whether we're applying useful techniques or using our garden as a guinea pig?

This book was created for those of you who don't buy what self-professed experts are selling just because everyone else does. It's for those of you who want the best for your garden but are skeptical of unproven claims. And it is especially for those of you who think it's wise to understand why and how something works before slathering it on the plants that took you so long to grow and that you take so much pride in caring for. For you there is good news. This book offers information on various products and practices that the gurus recommend, and it investigates these claims critically, sometimes with general knowledge, sometimes with scholarly articles, and sometimes with original research specifically designed to get to the truth. This book isn't intended to tell you how to garden. Rather, it investigates what the compounds on the garden center shelf or those that you make yourself in a home-brewed concoction will do to and for your plants. In the end, after perusing the pages herein, you will be able to distinguish between the garden remedies that work and those that are merely hearsay. What's more, you will be armed with a knowledge of the underlying principles behind each remedy's success or failure, allowing you to take a more objective and scientific approach to the advice you hear in the future.

The garden gurus and me

The first time I stood in front of a group of gardeners to speak about pesticides, I was asked a question about using a home-brewed remedy for controlling insects (I don't even remember which one). I froze. I was startled that someone would ask me about a home-brewed remedy when there were so many good commercial remedies out there. I was also embarrassed, as people with freshly minted Ph.D.s usually are when posed with a question they cannot answer relating to their subject area. I was especially embarrassed because, having graduate degrees in both entomology and horticulture, I thought I knew everything. Boy was I wrong. But that question was just the start of my encounters with homemade and unusual remedies for garden problems. I was, and still am, continually asked by master gardeners, homeowners, and students about the value of the tips and techniques they see on TV, on the Web, or in old books. As these questions come up, I do my best to answer them. Sometimes I succeed, and sometimes I don't. But when I don't, I have a new subject to research when I get back to the office. I wish it were possible to cover all the home-brewed helpers that are swimming around out there either on the internet, in magazines, or in books. Unfortunately this is impossible for obvious reasons.

The barrage of questions I am asked about remedies seems never ending, and although they come from a variety of sources, they most commonly originate from advice given by what I like to call "garden gurus." What is a garden guru? Well, to me a garden guru is a good (usually great) gardener who considers him- or herself something of an expert in most areas that have to do with gardening, who likes to give out information and recommendations, and, most importantly, who does not really understand the science behind the information or recommendations he or she is giving. Garden gurus are usually neighbors or gardening experts on TV. They are often home-taught wizards trying to teach us a thing or two about growing a plant without resorting to any of those recommendations that university professors think up. No way, they can get the same results with stuff right out of the cabinet! Truth be told, cabinet cures can actually work. But many have drawbacks, including being dangerous for the environment and dangerous to your plant's health. Here I will admit that I have been a garden guru, too. I have quickly given incorrect advice based on some harebrained notion from the top of my head rather than advice based on sound research. Let's face it: most of us have been a garden guru at one point or another in our lives, and those who claim they haven't are probably either lying or else they have never given gardening advice. I tend to be hard on the garden gurus (including myself) because I get tired of seeing the end results of their brand of advice, including burned leaves, black roots, and dead plants. Let me step back for a moment, however, and give these people some credit. While they may bring questionable practices to the table, they also provide excitement, energy, and creativity to the gardening world, something that cannot always be said for university professors like me.

As I traveled the road of becoming a professional teacher, researcher, and extension specialist, I have had the opportunity to meet many people who influenced my life in various ways, including Dan Horton, an entomology professor and extension specialist at the University of Georgia. Dan offered me insight into many areas, but the most important thing he ever said to me occurred one rainy afternoon when we had nothing to do but sit around and shoot the bull. "Jeff," he said, "extension is nothing more than the delivery of research-based information to those who can actually use it—don't make it more complicated than it is." To this day, I remember those words and try to follow his simple lesson.

Doing research is easy; getting it to the people who can actually use it is the tough part. This book attempts to deliver research-based information that has not been readily available to gardeners who are considering various garden remedies. It has been created for all of us who have either been gardening gurus or taken advice from them at one point or another in our lives and who want to evolve into informed gardeners.

A little bit about format

The products and practices in this book have been divided into four groups: fertilizers (chapter 2), products that affect water relations (chapter 3), a chapter on biostimulants (chapter 4), and pesticides and protectants (chapters 5–9). Each chapter includes entries for various products and remedies.

These entries have been divided into five sections: a brief introduction, a section on practice, a section on the theory behind the remedy, a section on the real story, and a section on what it all means to you. The introduction is just that, an introduction to the remedy in question and an explanation of what the remedy is used for. The section on practice describes how the remedy is used, and the section on theory provides some information on why the remedy should work. The information in these three sections comes from the people who sell or recommend the remedy. As a general rule, I have decided not to name the people making these claims. The recommendations are often made by many different sources, and the goal of evaluating various ingredients for plant growth and health is not to endorse or to denigrate any particular person, company, or product. Rather, the goal is to provide factual information. If you are curious and want to find out which companies and garden gurus recommend or sell particular products, then I suggest searching the internet, where you will quickly find out who is selling or recommending what.

The section covering the real story behind the various remedies is the most important part of each description. It examines data that has been collected by professional researchers. This data is extremely valuable for discovering how well something works and why. This section is not exhaustive and does not cover every facet of a product or remedy, but it does investigate the basic reasons why the remedy might or might not work. Additionally, for some products and practices where good research is lacking, I have undertaken small research projects to verify or elucidate the effects that the recommendations might have on a plant. In these situations I have done my best to provide a thorough and honest assessment of the results.

The final section discusses what the information means to you. It gives a summary of what a product or practice might do to or for a plant and in what situations it might be most useful, based on the research. The information offered here is in no way the final say on any of these remedies. Indeed, many of the remedies have not been sufficiently studied for anyone to make a final decision on their value in the garden. My goal is simply to give gardeners a better understanding of the science behind the practices. For quick reference, a rating of the usefulness of each product or practice is indicated by a row of flowerheads in the section "What it means to you." The ratings consider the benefits of a product and its dangers. Hence, a product that is supposed to kill insects may do a wonderful job of that, but if it also causes the leaves of most plants to burn and curl, then it will receive a low rating. In general the rating system can be interpreted as follows:

☘ Benefits are unlikely.

☘☘ Benefits, if any, are way out of line with claims.

☘☘☘ Benefits are likely under certain conditions, but not as good as most companies or garden gurus claim.

☘☘☘☘ Benefits are likely, under appropriate conditions, to at least come close to matching the claims of companies or garden gurus.

☘☘☘☘☘ Benefits are likely under most conditions if the product or remedy is used properly.

Classic concoctions

When I was younger one of my favorite pastimes was paging through old books and journals looking for interesting and forgotten techniques for growing plants. People are fascinated by past traditions and ideas and will sometimes try insane remedies just because they were once advertised as gems of ancient knowledge. Unfortunately for gardeners (or maybe fortunately as you read some recommendations!), many of the old practices pale in comparison to modern techniques. These old remedies still have historical interest, however, and can often give modern gardeners an insight into the prevailing ideas of their predecessors. Perhaps we may stop to think how our home-brewed remedies will look to future generations of gardeners. Any practices that have been around prior to 1950 are considered classic concoctions—regardless of their usefulness—and have been identified by the symbol.

Acknowledgments

A number of people helped to make this book possible. I would like to thank Janna Beckerman, Doug Foulk, Chad Giblin, Max Gibson, Hy Gillman, David Hanson, Suzanne Hardee-Gillman, Brian Horgan, Gary Johnson, Carl Rosen, Eric Zenner, and everyone else who put their efforts into editing, researching topics, or taking over some responsibilities for me so that

I had the time to complete this book. I would especially like to thank Chad Giblin for helping to conduct the research contained herein. In most cases in the text where I indicate that I conducted an experiment, it was with the help of someone else, and that someone was usually Chad. Finally, I would like to thank all the researchers who work in the applied plant sciences or in extension. It is truly you who made this book possible.

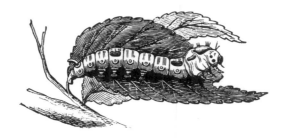

1

Basics

THE WORLD is full of the color green. Everywhere we look, from the city streets to the desert sands, there is plant life. No matter the situation, plants seem to grow and even to prosper despite the best efforts of people and geography. Yet we are not happy. If there is an oak in our backyard, we are disappointed if it is small; if there is a rose on our trellis, we are disappointed if it is not covered in bloom; if there is a spiraea on our patio and it is not covered in bright, new, colorful foliage, we are disappointed. We are, to steal a word from the psychology literature, optimizers. As gardeners we cannot stand the idea of a plant that does not reach its full potential. We want our plants to perform, and as plant lovers, we are willing to go to extreme lengths to get what we want—from applying hazardous chemicals to talking to them to applying odd concoctions of cleaners and intoxicants found in old storage cabinets because someone who may or may not have any experience with these products has recommended them. Surely, there is a better way to treat plants.

Nature is the best teacher of plant growth. Look at five different birch trees that were planted at the same time but in five different places, and you are likely to find quite a range of growth and health. This doesn't surprise even the most amateur gardener; after all, the five different locations offer five different types of soil, five different shade levels, five different drainage scenarios, and five different levels of nutrition. After investigating the trees and the sites on which they were planted, we can easily deduce the better conditions for the growth of that tree. This type of observation should guide us in arranging a setting that is conducive to growing plants, but it often does not. We thoughtlessly push plants into situations where they don't belong, moving them into colder, hotter, wetter, drier, shadier, sunnier, and just plain more inappropriate conditions. And what do we do if they don't perform the way we think they should? We apply more water, more fertilizer, more vitamins, more chemicals, and more misguided garden remedies until the plant either conforms to our will or dies trying. It is not wrong to try these solutions, but it is to our distinct advantage to understand the products we apply so that we will know how our plants will respond to them.

These modern times have yielded an incredible number of new products for increasing the growth of our plants, reducing the need to water, stimulating roots, and a myriad of other things. Many of them are good, and many are bad. Many of these products have not been sufficiently tested for us to have a really good sense of whether they work or not. But hey, who needs evidence that a product works in order to sell it? It's worth your time to figure out what a product is likely to do to your plants before you buy it. Some products may have a beneficial effect, some may do nothing, and some may actually be harmful. Naming all the gardening products in use today would be impossible. Fortunately, that is not necessary in order to understand which ones might be helpful for the garden—most of the products out there use the same active ingredients. Just look at the label of most fertilizers, pesticides, and other gardening concoctions, and you will find a list of the chemicals that may affect your plant, called "active ingredients." Look also at the ingredient list for the home-brewed remedies suggested by garden gurus. By matching the ingredients in these products and recipes with the information in this book, you can figure out what effects they are likely to have on plants before you risk their health and potentially your own.

Elements that affect plant growth and development

Before entering into a discussion of all the many and varied amendments for your garden, we must first understand the players. That is to say, it is important to understand what goes into growing a plant and how and why these things can affect a plant's growth. Only by understanding these basics can we understand how manipulating growing conditions can affect the growth and health of our plants. An incredible number of books out there provide this information in a more detailed fashion than is offered here, but for our purposes it is enough to understand the basics of plant growth and development.

Soil and media

All plants grow in some kind of soil or medium. The word *soil* usually refers to the naturally occurring substance in your yard or garden, and the word *media* (*medium*, singular) usually applies to substances placed in containers that do not include, or only include a small amount of, naturally occurring soil. Media typically include a large amount of such material as peat, composted pine bark, and rice hulls. The primary functions of soils and media, at least as far as your plants are concerned, are to hold plants upright and to hold water, air, and nutrients for the plants to use.

Soils have a number of characteristics that affect their ability to fulfill their primary functions. First, soil texture is important to a plant because it determines how much water and nutrition the soil can hold. Soils that contain a lot of sand will not hold much nutrition or much water but will drain quickly. Soils that contain a lot of clay will hold a great deal of water and nutrition but will not drain rapidly. An easy way to tell whether your soil is largely sand or clay is to get it wet and run your fingers through it. If the soil feels smooth, it is probably mostly clay. If it feels grainy, then it is probably mostly sand. To complicate the issue even more, most soils have organic matter in them. Organic matter is basically nothing more than decomposed plants and animals (compost is an example). Organic matter is generally beneficial to the soil because it is able to hold water and nutrients well, like clay, while also offering good drainage, like sand. Most media are made of organic matter of one form or another such as peat, composted bark, composted wood chips, and rice hulls to name just a few. These media components are usually chosen because of their ability to hold nutrients and water effectively while offering excellent drainage. Virtually every commercial planting medium that you can buy at garden centers has these qualities.

When a plant's roots are in a soil or medium, they tend to grow toward a particular balance of water and air. Yes, it's true; plant roots need air, too. In a highly clay soil this means that a plant's roots will congregate near the surface because, with the lack of drainage, there is not much air deep in the soil profile. Conversely, in a sandy soil that has excellent drainage, the plant's roots will need to go deeper to find sufficient water. If a plant is transplanted from a clay soil to a sandy soil or vice versa, all kinds of problems typically arise right off the bat because of the position of the roots at transplant and the position the roots would ideally like to have. Many people think they can cure these problems with special water-retention products or root-growth enhancers when they transplant. These products will be addressed later on—some have merits, but some are pretty useless.

Besides these properties, soils and media have another property that can profoundly affect a plant's ability to grow under certain conditions: pH. The pH of a planting medium is a measure of its acidity, and it determines the availability of nutrients that a plant needs in order to grow. A pH of 5.5 to 6.5 is typically considered best for the growth of most plants. One location where pH can affect the availability of nutrition is in the midwestern United States, where high pH soils are often found. In these high pH soils, iron and manganese, two nutrients that are essential to plant growth, are not available for many plants even though they may be in the soil. This causes a severe problem for plants such as blueberry, azalea, and rhododendron, which cannot obtain these nutrients at a high pH. A pH value that is too low (highly acid soils) can also cause problems. Appendix 1 details the best pH range for particular plants. Many of the products covered in this book, such as lime, chelates, and soil acidifiers, are produced to address these problems.

The easiest way to determine the properties of your soil is to submit a sample to your state extension service or another soil-testing lab. By having your soil checked, you will be able to choose plants that are appropriate for the location, and you will, hopefully, have little need for many of the practices mentioned in this book. Alternatively, there are do-it-yourself soil tests for sale at garden centers, and in general these tests work well but do not substitute for the more complete testing offered by state extension services.

Water

Soil is a good start, but dry soil alone will not grow plants. Soils need to be able to hold water to support plant life. Watering, though apparently easy, is difficult to do properly. Ensuring the roots are neither drying nor drowning is an underappreciated art. Overwatering is just as dangerous as underwatering, and unfortunately, they share the same symptoms (leaves droop and turn brown at the edges). Some general rules about watering are worth noting. First, soil type has a lot to do with how often watering needs to be done. Sandy soils need frequent watering, while clay soils and soils high in organic matter usually need less-frequent watering. Because containers have such a small amount of media to actually hold the water, they will usually need to be watered more often than plants in a landscape. It is much better to apply water over an extended period of time than to apply it in a short period of time. When water is applied quickly the soil particles do not have sufficient time to absorb the water and much of it is lost. When water is applied slowly the soil has a better chance to absorb it. This principle is easily demonstrated with two dry sponges of the same size (and from the same package if possible) and a small glass of water. Quickly dump the water over the first sponge (make the application in less than a second). How much of the water was absorbed? How wet is the sponge? Now add the same amount of water from the same glass to the second sponge over a longer period of time. Take 30 seconds or so. How wet is this sponge? This quick example teaches us much about proper watering; namely, if you want to water something well you need to be patient.

But why does soil or media need to be watered at all? How does water leave these substances? Water can be lost from media or soil in two ways. The first is water loss directly from the medium or soil itself. This happens when water either evaporates or drains through the substance, and it occurs regardless of whether or not a plant is growing in the soil. The second way a soil or medium could lose water is through the plant. Plants take up water and incorporate it into their cells, but they also lose a certain amount of water to transpiration. Transpiration is somewhat similar to an animal's sweating—the plant has pores from which water can be lost to evaporation. This water loss is necessary for plants' physiological processes, such as the movement of nutrients in a plant's vascular system.

Most of the water-related products and practices covered in this book have one of two goals. The first is to increase the water-holding capacity of the soil or media, and the second is to block the plant's pores to prevent transpiration and hence reduce water loss. Both of these practices have merit on paper, but they may need some tweaking in practice as we will see later.

Nutrients

Plants need certain elements to grow. These elements are present in the soil, and when water is added they dissolve (to some extent) and become available for the plant to take up through its roots. The elements necessary for plant growth include boron, calcium, carbon, chlorine, copper, hydrogen, iron, magnesium, manganese, molybdenum, nitrogen, oxygen, phosphorus, potassium, sulfur, and zinc (sodium, silicon, and some others may also provide benefits to plants in some situations). Carbon, oxygen, and hydrogen are available in the air and water, so we don't often consider these elements when we talk about plant nutrition. Calcium, magnesium, nitrogen, phosphorus, potassium, and sulfur are required at higher levels than other nutrients and are usually called macronutrients. The other elements are considered micronutrients because they are needed in lower concentrations than the macronutrients. If any of these elements are not present, the plant will become sick and eventually die. Most soils contain the elements that support plant life; if they didn't the earth wouldn't have forests. However, plants usually grow better, or at least more quickly, when additional nutrition is offered to them.

In order to deliver nutrients to plants, people created fertilizers. Fertilizers are nothing more than substances that can be added to the soil around a plant (or in some cases to the plant itself) that will deliver nutrients that the plant needs. Fertilizers have taken on a life of their own. They can be applied in a variety of ways, such as liquid or granular, and provide a variety of nutrients in a variety of different concentrations, such as high nitrogen, low nitrogen, high phosphorus, or low phosphorus. Fertilizers can be organic or synthetic, and yes, too much of any fertilizer leads to injury and even death for the plant. Fertilizers are enough to make someone's head swim, but they can impact the growth and health of your plants. It is worth spending the time to understand them so you can have the best garden possible.

Plant hormones

Plants have hormones just like people do. Hormones are not nutritional and don't need to be acquired from the soil to promote growth. Rather, hormones are chemicals a plant produces naturally that signal the plant to do something, such as cease growth, drop leaves, produce flowers, or elongate. There are five basic plant hormones: abscisic acid, auxins, cytokinins, ethylene, and gibberellins, but other compounds have also been shown to act in a hormonal way on plants. Humans have manipulated plant hormones in a variety of ways to try to get plants to do what we want them to do, and a number of commercial products take advantage of plants' responses to various chemicals.

Auxins are the hormones that are most commonly manipulated by humans. In a nutshell, auxins stimulate growth. They are naturally present at the growing points of plants, such as at the tips of leaves, roots, and stems. By placing artificial auxins on various points of the plant, including cuttings of roots or stems, researchers and chemical companies hope to stimulate root growth. This can be useful for plant propagation or for stimulating root growth during transplanting.

Cytokinins, gibberellins, ethylene, and abscisic acid are less commercially valuable, although there are some products that utilize these hormones. Cytokinins are sometimes sold to improve blossom set and fruit yield; gibberellins are sometimes used to increase fruit size as well as to produce fruit without seeds; ethylene is sometimes used to promote leaf or fruit drop at the end of the year. These hormones are classified as commercial pesticides and are covered in chapter 9.

Pests

Most pests can be categorized into one of three varieties: insects, diseases, or weeds. Chemicals used to control any of these are generally called pesticides, a term that is often misinterpreted as referring specifically to insect-control agents. Pesticides can fall under numerous categories, most notably insecticides (for controlling insects), fungicides (for controlling fungal diseases), and herbicides (for controlling weeds).

Pests usually do one of three things that make us unhappy: kill plants, slow plant growth, or make plants look unsightly. Unfortunately, people often think that if their plant looks at all unsightly or grows even a little bit more slowly than their neighbor's, then there must be a problem. This is the furthest thing from the truth. While some pests certainly can and do kill, most pests cause just a small amount of damage and then move on.

Insects need to eat, and diseases need to infect to survive. They eat and infect the trees, shrubs, flowers, and grasses in our yards, but most pests don't kill plants for a very simple ecological reason. If they killed all the plants, then they would have nothing to eat or infect in the future. Besides, most plants are prepared to be attacked by insects and disease. Most trees and shrubs can actually lose 20 or even 30 percent of their leaf area without suffering a severe reduction in growth. The same applies to the effects of weeds. Without weeds our plants will certainly grow faster, but the fact is that trees and shrubs are adapted to living with weeds. If they couldn't live with weeds they would never have survived in nature. I'm not saying you shouldn't treat for the pests you see. Indeed, if I had a tree with 30 percent of its leaves missing, I would surely try to get rid of the pest. I do mulch my trees to get rid of weeds and achieve the best growth possible. What I am saying is that, for good or for ill, most of us tend to be more aggressive in trying to control pests than we have to be.

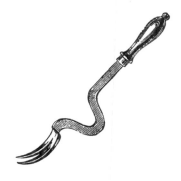

2

Fertilizers and Other Soil and Media Amendments

MAKING A SOIL or medium just right for our plants is a common goal of gardeners, but it sounds a great deal easier than it is. On garden-shop shelves, in gardening books, and on gardening shows, we see countless products and suggestions that are supposed to make our soil or media better for our plants in one way or another. The benefits offered by these remedies can range from altering the pH of the soil to conditioning it to adding nutrients such as iron or sulfur. Many of these products and suggestions are helpful, but many aren't. Indeed, some are incredibly dangerous to plants.

All things that can be added to a soil or medium fall under the amendment category. Fertilizers are nothing more than a type of amendment that adds nutrients. The amendments in this chapter include many things you might add to a soil or medium, with the exception of amendments intended to alter the water relations of a plant or to work as a biostimulant—those will be addressed in chapter 3 and chapter 4.

Fertilizers are by far the most common type of amendment (besides water!). They come in a wide variety of forms that may or may not be appropriate for you, depending on the situation in which your plants are growing. The most interesting types of fertilizer, at least to me, are those fertilizers advertised by garden gurus. These include things like beer, molasses, soda, and many other items that we think of as food for people rather than for plants. While researching this book, I came across such an incredible number of recommendations for these types of fertilizer that I simply could not cover them all. That wasn't much of a problem because there is really very little involved in understanding why foods that are good for us are also good for plants. When we eat food, we absorb proteins, carbohydrates, and fats. Plants generally don't absorb these compounds, but they do absorb the things that these foods are made of when they break down, including nitrogen, phosphorus, potassium, calcium, and all the other nutrients essential for plant life. Think of it this way. Most food we eat was once a living thing. That thing needed nutrients to live just as you do and just as a plant does. When that living thing died it didn't lose the nutrition it had absorbed during its life; rather, that nutrition was stored and can be transferred to another living creature, through eating in the case of humans or, in the case of plants, through allowing that once-living thing to decompose near its roots.

Ammonia, a quick and easy way to misapply fertilizer 🌱

Ammonia is sold in grocery stores as a cleaning compound, but this home-brewed helper is widely recommended by garden gurus and do-it-yourself wizards as the greatest fertilizer since cow dung. Homemade-fertilizer aficionados have been using "spirits of ammonia" since at least the 1800s, and there seems to be no slowing them down today. But why do we use something specially designed to clean floors as a homemade fertilizer? While ammonia is indeed a type of nitrogen, which microbes in the soil can convert into a form that plants can use, that doesn't explain why this potentially damaging chemical is so widely recommended.

The practice

Ammonia is commonly added to water to serve as a source of nitrogen for plants. Some garden gurus even recommend adding ammonia to regular fertilizers such as Miracle-Gro. (Why would you bother adding this stuff to Miracle-Gro, something that already has plenty of nitrogen in it?—I can't make sense of this one.) Recommendations vary from a few tablespoons per gallon of water to a few cups per gallon. If you're looking for old recommendations Anne Hale, a 19th-century gardener, recommended using a 2- or 3-ounce bottle of spirits of ammonia dissolved in a large pail of water as a stimulant for flowers (1871).

The theory

Ammonia is composed, primarily, of nitrogen. Nitrogen is good for plants if it is offered at an appropriate dose. Those who recommend using ammonia as a fertilizer believe this chemical can deliver nitrogen in a way that will help your plants to grow.

The real story

Homemade-fertilizer suggestions on the Web or in gardeners' how-to books recommend applying various quantities of ammonia to your garden or houseplant. These concoctions are reported to offer amazing growth. Unfortunately, you rarely see the author of these concoctions identify the concentration of ammonia in the product that they use. The problem, you see, is that the ammonia you buy in the store is actually a gas (the ammonia itself) dissolved in a liquid (water). This solution may contain anywhere from 3 to 10 percent ammonia. If you don't know the concentration of ammonia the garden guru used, then you are flying blind and likely to over- or under fertilize your plants, perhaps adding over three times more nitrogen than the author of the recipe did! Besides, many of the recommendations suggest using a hose-end sprayer but fail to indicate the calibration. Hose-end sprayers are not all adjusted to deliver their mixtures in the same concentration. They could apply 1 part fertilizer with anywhere from 16 to 80 parts water, or even a little more. This is bad news. If you don't know the dilution your sprayer makes, you are in danger of overapplying fertilizer, and an over-application of fertilizer can lead to some pretty-sick plants. But over-application of fertilizer is actually just the beginning of the problems with ammonia. We haven't even looked at the chemistry of the ammonia itself.

Household ammonia, created and formulated to clean floors, is made of a type of nitrogen that can be quite toxic to plants. Again, ammonia is a gas dissolved in water. After it dissolves, the gas combines with the water to form something called aqueous ammonia and something else called ammonium and hydroxide ions. Ammonium ions are useful as a fertilizer, but aqueous ammonia is toxic to seedlings at concentrations as low as 3.5 parts per million (Bennett and Adams 1970). The amount of aqueous ammonia that will be in your fertilizer solution is highly dependent on the pH of the water you are mixing your household ammonia with. If the pH of that water is over 7 then watch out! You are going to be releasing all kinds of aqueous ammonia. If you have a water pH in the acid range, there will be much less aqueous ammonia released—unless your soil is alkaline, in which case you're back to square one. What's that? You don't know the pH of your water or soil? Then you shouldn't even remotely consider using ammonia.

What it means to you ❀

Homemade fertilizers based on ammonia are not a good idea if you don't know what you're doing, and they're not a great idea even if you do know what you're doing. They are not that much cheaper than commercial fertilizers, and they have the potential to seriously damage your plants if used incorrectly.

Analyzing the ever-changing fertilizer analysis ⚘

Ever since the 1940s, when individual states passed laws requiring fertilizer companies to disclose nutrition information on their products' labels, companies have been altering the amount of nutrients in their products to try to encourage sales.

Fertilizers usually contain three primary elements, nitrogen, phosphorus, and potassium, and are differentiated by the ratio of these elements to one another; this ratio is called the analysis. The analysis of most common fertilizers includes three numbers and is usually displayed prominently on the front or rear label of the bag or container. These numbers indicate the percentage of nitrogen (N), phosphorus (expressed as P_2O_5), and potassium (expressed as K_2O) that a fertilizer delivers. That phosphorus and potassium are expressed as P_2O_5 and K_2O may seem a little silly, especially since there is rarely any K_2O or P_2O_5 in the fertilizer at all, but all fertilizers follow this blueprint so it is easy to compare one fertilizer to the next. For the sake of convenience I will refer to these elements simply as N (nitrogen), P (phosphorus), and K (potassium), meaning that a fertilizer with an analysis of 12-2-12 contains 12 percent N, 2 percent P, and 12 percent K.

There are many fertilizer analyses, some with high nitrogen, some with high phosphorus, some with high potassium, and some with a mixture, and each is supposedly formulated for specific plants and specific needs. But are these combinations useful tools that help us to fertilize our plants appropriately, or are they gimmicks that lead us to buy more products than we actually need?

The practice

If you search hard enough, you will find fertilizers with almost any type of analysis you could want. One analysis is supposed to be better than another for starting seeds, another is better for blooming plants, and so on. There is no doubt that altering analyses is good for fertilizer producers.

The theory

There are three basic reasons why fertilizer companies offer more than one analysis. The first is that not all plants are created equal—different plants require different quantities of different nutrients. The second is that at different stages of a plant's life, it requires different levels of nutrition. For example, it is commonly believed that when seeds are sown, a fertilizer high in phosphorus (such as 10-26-10) is better than a fertilizer high in nitrogen (such as 22-3-3). Finally, companies offer different analyses because of the physical limitations of concentrating or altering natural fertilizers. It is not possible to change the analysis of natural fertilizers, such as bat guano, to any great degree.

The real story

Before we begin to discuss the benefits of fertilizer analyses, it is important to understand that we are discussing the ratio of nutrients to one another rather than the actual amount of nitrogen, phosphorus, or potassium found in the fertilizer itself. Any two fertilizers with the same ratio of nitrogen-phosphorus-potassium can offer the same nutrition. For example, any fertilizer with a nitrogen-phosphorus-potassium ratio of 1-2-1 (such as 10-20-10, 5-10-5, and 6-12-6) can be applied so that 1 pound of nitrogen, 2 pounds of phosphorus, and 1 pound of potassium are released per 1000 square feet. The benefit that the fertilizer producer is trying to sell you is derived primarily from the ratio of nutrients to one another. Another important thing to remember is that, while nitrogen needs to be reapplied year to year, or even month to month, phosphorus and potassium tend to stick around for quite a long time and do not need to be reapplied nearly as frequently. Hence, a single application of nitrogen, phosphorus, and potassium will supply the soil with phosphorus and potassium for much longer than it will supply nitrogen.

Nitrogen is the most important element to a plant's growth, and in most situations the amount of nitrogen available is what determines how well the plant will grow. Some plants, however, have the ability to thrive under conditions of high nitrogen while others do not. Poinsettias, for example, can use high concentrations of nitrogen, while tulips must be fertilized only lightly with nitrogen (Nelson 2003). Likewise, certain crops, such as fruits and nuts, have high requirements for potassium because they take more potassium from the soil than they do any other element (Westwood 1993). So it is easy to see that for heavy nitrogen feeders, a high analysis of nitrogen is appropriate (something like 20-5-5), and that for fruit and nut producers, fertilizers with a high analysis of potassium (something like 20-10-20) are appropriate. The plants will use up the nutrients they need more quickly than the nutrients they don't need, and applying high levels of nutrients they don't need results in a lot of wasted nutrition.

Besides differing fertilizer requirements for different plants, there are other reasons to alter fertilizer analyses. A huge number of fertilizers out there are supposed to promote an increase in bloom and are supposed to be good "starter fertilizers" for plants that have been recently planted. These fertilizers generally include a huge proportion of phosphorus, such as 10-52-10. This may have some benefits, depending on the type of plant and its stage of life. For example, grass likes to have some extra phosphorus available when it is just starting out but doesn't need much after it has become established (Christians 1998). Phosphorus is immobile in the soil, and young plants like to have phosphorus "bottle fed" to them because they do not have a large enough root system to gather this nutrient for themselves. Later in life, however, plants do not need higher levels of phosphorus, so any extra that is applied either hangs out in the soil waiting to be used at some later time or else gets washed into streams and lakes, causing pollution.

If we take a look at the amount of phosphorus in plant leaf tissue, something that has been done for thousands of plants, we see that there is usually less phosphorus in plants than the two other nutrients on the fertilizer label, nitrogen and potassium. And there is usually more calcium, magnesium, and even sulfur in plant tissues than phosphorus (Mills and Jones 1996).

Are you starting to get the impression that these high phosphorus fertilizers may not be all they're cracked up to be? But what about claims that high phosphorus fertilizers can increase bloom and stimulate rooting? These are claims that I see again and again, but they really aren't supported by the literature.

To check out the claims that phosphorus can promote rooting in recently planted shrubs, I performed a study in which I transplanted roses, lilacs, and potentillas from smaller containers into larger containers. While transplanting, I left the roots in the tight mass that was formed from the first container rather than teasing them out as is recommended for a newly planted shrub. The soil in the second containers included either no phosphorus, a moderate amount of phosphorus, or an extremely high amount of phosphorus. After one season of growth the plants were removed from the larger containers, and the new roots that had spread from the root ball and into the media were carefully removed and weighed. If phosphorus indeed allows the plant to produce more roots, then we should have been able to measure this by a greater weight of roots in the containers with higher phosphorus. We did not see this at all and, indeed, most scientists who do studies like this get results similar to ours. To quote Timothy Broschat and Kimberly Klock-Moore (2000) of the University of Florida, "Most container grown plants require only minimal amounts of P for optimal growth and . . . applications of high P fertilizers will not promote either root or shoot growth in plants as popularly believed." Although these scientists were talking specifically about plants grown in containers, there is little reason to believe that their statement isn't equally true in the garden.

There is little evidence that phosphorus promotes flowering—unless a soil is quite deficient in this nutrient. In fact, an old friend of mine, Donglin Zhang, an associate professor at the University of Maine, recently found that fanflower has reduced growth and flowering when fed high levels of phosphorus (Zhang et al. 2004). Naturally, if no phosphorus is present, there will be a problem. In that case phosphorus needs to be added, but as long as some phosphorus is present, there is little reason to believe that additional phosphorus will increase bloom or fruit set. But what about nitrogen? High levels of nitrogen have long been known to promote vegetative growth at the expense of flowering and fruiting (Kenrick 1833). You can easily demonstrate this to yourself by applying two or three times the recommended dose of nitrogen to your tomatoes and seeing how long it takes for them to flower when compared to tomatoes fertilized with the proper amount of nitrogen. Adding a lot of nitrogen, or a lot of phosphorus, is not a great idea if you want to stimulate flowers.

It would seem that fertilizer analyses really do make a difference. But wait! We are forgetting something. What happens to plants that never receive fertilizer? When plants grow in the wild they seldom, if ever, are fertilized with optimal amounts of nitrogen, phosphorus, or potassium, yet they function well enough to produce beautiful floral displays, reproduce themselves, and grow to fantastic sizes. So what does this mean? It means that plants are wired to accept a wide range of nutrients and will usually grow and be at least somewhat productive even without additional fertilizer. In fact, in some studies, additions of fertilizer do not increase the growth of plants (Paine et al. 1992).

What it means to you ❀❀❀❀

Claims made by fertilizer companies about particular fertilizer analyses are usually basically true, with the exception of the claim that adding large quantities of phosphorus promotes blooms or stimulates roots. However, the claims are usually out of line with the magnitude of the effect that different fertilizers will have, unless your soil is completely devoid of nutrients (something that is rare). Higher levels of nitrogen will grow plants more effectively than high levels of other elements (be careful of overfertilizing, though). Phosphorus and potassium are needed, especially potassium for fruits and vegetables, and you will benefit from having the levels of these element tested in your soil and adding more if they are lacking. If they are present at moderate levels, though, you will not see big gains in plant growth or health by adding more. Because these elements are relatively immobile in soil, a few applications of phosphorus and potassium may last for years, especially if you have a good soil rich in organic matter. If your soil is sandy these elements are likely to last for a shorter period of time. If you see problems with plant growth and you have been applying a fertilizer that includes nitrogen, phosphorus, and potassium at any concentration, then the source of the problem is much more likely to be improper watering, a lack of micronutrients, an inappropriate pH, or even overfertilization, than a deficiency of any of these three nutrients.

Beer as a fertilizer

Among the wackier gardening advice, some recommended aids are ubiquitous. Beer, used as a fertilizer, is a prime example. While poring through old gardening literature, I am always on the lookout for beer, maybe because I want to find out where the garden gurus came up with the idea, or maybe just because I like beer. Interestingly enough, beer really doesn't appear in the old gardening books very much at all, except for hops. In 1890 Peter Henderson recommended refuse hops from breweries as an excellent fertilizer, 50 percent more valuable than stable manure. So if you live near a brewery and have access to discarded hops, these might be an excellent addition to your garden. In terms of beer—well, let's find out.

The practice

Beer is usually recommended for the lawn, but it is also recommended for the vegetable or flower garden. Recommendations are usually for about a tablespoon of beer added to every gallon of water, but they can include concentrations of up to a full can of beer, undiluted, for a small yard area.

The theory

I think the main reason people recommend beer is that it sounds avant-garde. Their explanations of why it works, however, offer a different story. Generally, beer is recommended as a source of vitamins and minerals that your plant needs for healthy and quick growth. It has also been suggested that beer offers food for beneficial microorganisms, such as bacteria, and that it may even add some of these beneficial microorganisms itself.

The real story

There is very little information anywhere on why adding beer to plants might result in increased health and growth, so it seems odd at first glance that anyone ever thought of using it. A closer investigation of what is in beer, however, will provide some insight as to why it might, just might, be beneficial to a plant under certain conditions. Beer contains water, carbon dioxide, ethanol (the alcohol that inebriates us), a wide variety of carbohydrates (sugars) that make the beer taste good, a small quantity of protein (which contains nitrogen), and a few other things, such as trace elements, in very small quantities.

First things first, the water in beer is neither here nor there. If the beer is being applied with water, as is usually the case, then the water in the beer is simply along for the ride. On the other hand, if the beer is the only source of water for a plant, then having it is certainly better than dying of drought. Likewise, carbon dioxide is unlikely to have an effect on the plant, as there is already substantial carbon dioxide in the air. Ethanol is not helpful to plant growth; in fact, ethanol can be quite detrimental, causing plant burn and even death. That leaves us with carbohydrates and protein. Various carbohydrates, also known as sugars, have been shown to be taken up by the roots of plants (Begna et al. 2002; Saftner and Wyse 1984). Carbohydrates are the building blocks of plants, so these additional carbohydrates could help, but protein is the more likely answer as to why beer might increase plant growth and health, if indeed it does. After all, protein includes nitrogen, the fertilizer component that is most likely to result in a growth response from the plant. Beer contains about 6 grams of protein in every liter (about ¼ gallon) (Gorinstein et al. 1999), which, while not a huge amount, could certainly be helpful if no other source of nitrogen is available. Besides the protein, other nutrients your plants need are present in beer, such as iron, copper, and zinc (Wyrzykowska et al. 2001), but the concentrations of these are probably too low to help plant growth much unless they are completely absent in the soil. So beer does contain some nutrients that could help plant growth, but it also contains ethanol, which should inhibit plant growth.

Does beer really encourage plant growth? What about the growth of bacteria that might be beneficial to plant roots? These questions are difficult to answer with the available research because very few people have actually taken the time to compare the growth of plants treated with beer to plants not treated with beer. Fortunately, your intrepid narrator has tested a variety of beer on the growth of a garden favorite, the butterfly bush. These tests were conducted in hydroponic conditions to avoid the influence of other factors in the soil. The beers that were tested included a light beer (Michelob Light), a stout (Guinness), and an alcohol-free beer (Sharps). Beer was added to water in hydroponic tubs, along with a low concentration of liquid fertilizer (similar to what would be found in a good, unfertilized, garden soil). Six plants were grown with each type of beer at a concentration of either 6 ounces or 12 ounces in a 5½-gallon tub. We also ran a control (a hydroponic set up with the fertilizer but without the beer) and an alcohol test (we added to the fertilizer as much ethanol as is found in 12 ounces of Michelob Light). Over time, notes were taken on the growth of plants.

The results of this experiment were clear cut: alcohol is bad for plant growth, beer with alcohol is bad for plant growth, and beer without alcohol is bad for plant growth, although small amounts of alcohol-free beer didn't do any major harm. In short, the best plants were those that didn't have anything besides a small amount of fertilizer added. (More fertilizer probably would have increased growth more, but since the experiment was conducted to look at beer, we didn't examine this.) What about beneficial bacteria? Well, most of the plants that suffered did indeed have a huge amount of bacteria around their roots. If these bacteria were beneficial, though, we would have expected some result other than stunting and death. The problem here is that the garden gurus assume that because beer increases bacterial growth it must increase the number of beneficial bacteria; they forget all about the bad bacteria. Based on our experiment, bad bacteria seem to enjoy beer just as much as good bacteria, or maybe even more.

There is one thing that some people claim about beer, however, that our research did not investigate: the addition of beneficial organisms. I have heard garden gurus claim that the yeast in beer makes it a valuable addition to soils because it speeds the composting of dead organic material, such as thatch, in the yard or garden. This is hard to believe because most commercial beer goes through pasteurization or some other sterilization process, such as filtration. There should be almost no living yeast, or other microorganisms for that matter, in most beers. Finally, even if the beer did have some live yeast left in it, yeast is extremely common. You could not prevent yeast from reaching your garden even if you wanted to; hence, applying beer to your yard or garden to introduce this or other microorganisms is a waste of time.

What it means to you ✽

Beer is better consumed than applied to your garden. Although many reasons were given above as to why beer might be beneficial to plant growth, the fact remains that in our experiment it was, in fact, harmful. Adding small quantities of beer to a garden probably wouldn't be as detrimental to plants as our experiment concluded, but why risk it? A huge number of lawn fertilizers are formulated especially for your garden and grass. If you care enough about your garden to have read this section, then you probably care enough to take the time to fertilize and water properly. If you fertilize and water properly there is no reason to believe that beer will provide any additional benefits besides allowing you to appear avant-garde.

Buttermilk and other high-protein foods

A few recommendations for adding people foods to your soil are guaranteed to give your plants a boost. These recommendations are for foods such as milk and gelatin that are high in protein. Proteins are made of amino acids that, in turn, are full of nitrogen, which plants love.

The practice

A few of the most common high-protein foods recommended as home-brewed helpers by garden experts include gelatin, buttermilk, and powdered milk. There is huge variation in the recommendations of concentration and amount of the various milk products to use when fertilizing, but most milk-based fertilizer recipes settle on about 1 part liquid milk added to 4 parts water and usually recommend that 1 to 2 cups of this mixture be applied to a medium-sized potted plant or garden shrub. Unflavored gelatin, another high-nitrogen people food, is often recommended at a concentration of one packet of unflavored gelatin dissolved in 1 cup of water, to be applied to a potted plant or a small garden space.

The theory

Foods that are high in protein contain a high concentration of nitrogen. In theory, the nitrogen is released and becomes available to plants as the food breaks down in the soil.

The real story

There is no doubt that high-protein food contains nitrogen. The question is whether this nitrogen is appropriate for plants and can do the same job as commercial fertilizers. To test how well high-nitrogen people food works as a fertilizer, I decided to compare buttermilk to a commercial slow-release fertilizer. I used buttermilk because, as anyone who has ever opened a broken refrigerator knows, milk goes bad quickly, decomposing into its constituent elements, including nitrogen. In this experiment I grew three sets of tomato plants: one with buttermilk as a fertilizer, one with no fertilizer added, and one with a slow-release synthetic fertilizer. The plants fertilized with buttermilk were treated to about 2 cups of a mixture of 1 part buttermilk added to 4 parts water. The buttermilk and synthetic fertilizers were only applied once, at the time the seeds were planted. I added nothing else, besides water, to the tomato seeds over the course of this experiment; no fertilizers, no biostimulants, nothing. I planted about eight tomato seeds per container and thinned them to four plants per container soon after the seeds germinated and before any size differences were evident. Just 2 weeks after the tomato seeds germinated, the plants that were fertilized with the slow-release fertilizer were clearly larger and stronger than the plants that were fertilized with the buttermilk, which were, in turn, larger and stronger than the plants that received no fertilizer. As time went on, these differences became more and more evident. This experiment shows something most of you probably already know. Commercial fertilizers are better for plants than buttermilk, but buttermilk is far better than nothing.

Though high-nitrogen people food might not always be the best choice for delivering nitrogen to plants, especially potted plants, where nutrition can be quickly washed through the pot, it is certainly a very useful constituent of compost. Compost that has a wide variety of constituents, including a healthy dose of high-nitrogen people food, will provide nutrition to plants that renders fertilizing less necessary in a garden setting.

Nitrogen-containing foods do tend to be more effective in a garden setting (either in compost or alone) than in containers because a healthy soil is better able to hold nutrients than media in containers, which are constantly subjected to water drenches that drive nutrients out. Also keep in mind that plants in a garden are able to spread their roots out over a larger area than they can in a container, allowing them to search for nutrients, including nitrogen, more effectively.

What it means to you ✽✽✽✽

Milk comes from a cow to provide nutrition for a calf, not a plant. High-nitrogen people food certainly contains nitrogen, which plants love. This nutrient can be delivered to a plant through buttermilk, gelatin, a ham sandwich, or even a peanut candy bar, but a commercial fertilizer has an advantage in that you can be pretty sure you are giving your plant an appropriate dose of nutrition for their needs, not to mention you avoid wasting food. So why am I giving this stuff a four? The key is that it can deliver nitrogen to your plants. If you have been careful to put high-nitrogen food waste in your compost, then you are making good use of these foods and saving yourself money in the long run. But if you are purchasing buttermilk or other high-nitrogen food items specifically to fertilize plants, this practice will cost you more over the course of a year than using commercial fertilizers.

Chelates

Chelates are chemicals present in Sequestrene, ericaceous plant foods, liquid iron, and other products intended for use on plants that prefer acid soils or are very nutrient deficient. These chemicals are bound to elements, such as iron, and allow those elements to be more easily taken up by plants, offering a quick fix of nutrients. Chelates can offer nutrients over a pH range that is much greater than normal, and they are most commonly used for plants in soils that are too alkaline (the pH is too high) for them.

The practice

Chelates are administered to plants by applying them either directly to the surrounding soil or to the leaves. They contain a number of nutrients, most notably iron and manganese, which are lacking because the plant has been growing in an inappropriate site. Chelates usually move rapidly through soil, so recommendations often indicate that these products should be administered frequently.

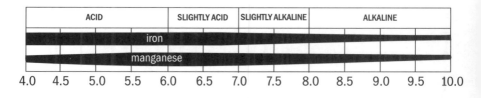

Figure 1. The relative availability of iron and manganese at different pH levels. High pH is the primary reason that people use chelates.

The theory

By binding elements such as iron and manganese to chemicals that will deliver them to a plant despite variations in pH, these products are supposed to make nutrients available to plants that would normally not be able to take them up because of soil conditions.

The real story

Chelates do make elements more available to plants under pH conditions that would normally inhibit the uptake of these elements (Yunta et al. 2003). Iron chelates are the most common and are especially useful for plants such as azaleas, rhododendrons, and blueberries that have been planted in soils that are too alkaline for them. Chelates tend not to last very long, and though some research on citrus has shown chelates may need to be applied every 4 weeks or so (Banuls et al. 2003), how often these products need to be reapplied is likely to vary widely based on the plants that are being treated, the chelates that are being used, weather conditions, and other factors.

What it means to you ❀❀❀❀

The best choice, of course, is to plant plants that prefer more-acidic soils in more-acidic soils. If you just can't live without your acid-loving plant and you live in a place where it is impossible to find acidic soils, chelates will supply the nutrients, primarily iron, that these misplaced souls are lacking. Chelates will probably need to be applied at least once every month or two to keep your plants healthy. A better long-term solution is to use soil acidifiers, such as sulfur, so that the soil itself can offer the proper nutrients to your plants. There is usually nothing wrong with applying sulfur at the same time as treating a plant with a chelate so that you can get the short term effect of the chelate along with the long term effect of the sulfur, but it is best to apply them separately to avoid possible chemical reactions.

Coffee grounds

Coffee grounds are the part of the coffee that is left when you're done brewing. Most home compost piles include some coffee grounds, but some people recommend sprinkling coffee grounds from fresh-made coffee right onto the soil near your plants. Can your plants benefit from this little morning pick-me-up the same way that we do?

The practice

Though organic gardeners and garden gurus seem to agree that this stuff is the cat's meow, recommendations for the application of coffee grounds tend to be inexact. Most recipes recommend simply sprinkling some around your plants.

The theory

Coffee grounds are organic matter and will break down, just like any compost, into their component elements, which could be beneficial for plant growth. Coffee also may contain chemicals that inhibit weed growth. Additionally, if coffee's ability to give you heartburn is any indication, it ought to be able to acidify the soil, too.

The real story

When a living thing dies and breaks down it gives off nutrients stored during its life. Coffee grounds contain about 2 percent nitrogen, 0.3 percent phosphorus, and 0.3 percent potassium (Stephens 1994), as well as some micronutrients. So why separate coffee grounds but not banana peels or ham sandwiches? Quite simply, coffee grounds are different from banana peels and other foods we might decide to put on the ground where our plants are growing. Researchers have looked extensively at these little bits of organic material and have found that they can have effects on your crop beyond those of a simple fertilizer.

Different plants seem to respond differently to the addition of coffee grounds to their soil or media. Some plants, such as lettuce, seem to benefit from coffee ground–amended soil quite a bit; some plants, such as alfalfa, seem to benefit very little; and some plants, such as ryegrass, wheat, and tomato, actually seem to be negatively affected (Kitou and Yoshida 1997). The negative impact may be caused by chemicals in the coffee, called allelopathic chemicals, which actually inhibit the growth of some plants (Kitou and Okuno 1999). Nonetheless, it seems that, at least for some plants, coffee grounds aren't too bad unless they're fresh, in which case there is a possibility the grounds will tie up nitrogen the plant might like to use itself (Waka-sawa et al. 1998). This makes sense because fresh vegetable matter (that's what coffee grounds are) actually tends to absorb more nitrogen than it gives off. Microbes use the nitrogen as fuel to break down the complex organic material into simpler sugars. Only after the vegetable matter decomposes for a period of time does it release nutrients instead of absorbing them.

Though I have read claims stating that once coffee is brewed all the acids are drawn out, research shows otherwise. European researchers have found that coffee residues do seem to affect the pH of the media they are mixed with. This may well offer some benefit for acid-loving plants (Reyes-Hernandez et al. 2002). Applying coffee grounds to the top of media or soil is less likely to affect its pH. Coffee itself has a pH of about 5 to 5.5 right out of the cup.

What it means to you ❀❀❀

Spreading coffee grounds around plants isn't a bad idea, but expecting them to affect pH to any great extent without incorporating them into the soil or media probably isn't realistic. Stick with the other soil acidifiers. It is possible that the allelopathic chemicals present in coffee may inhibit weed growth around your plants, which would surely help, and there is no doubt that the nutrients the grounds give off as they break down will benefit your plants. Fresh coffee grounds probably won't affect your plants' uptake of nitrogen too much unless you incorporate them into your soil. This is a bad idea not only because the coffee grounds might tie up nitrogen but also because the allelopathic chemicals you may be adding can't tell the difference between the plants you want to grow and plants you want to kill. For the same reason, pouring old coffee from a pot onto your plants isn't the greatest of ideas either (even though it might lower the pH of your soil).

Compost ☘

Compost is dead plant (and animal) materials that are decomposed, or decomposing, because of the microbes that are eating it. In fact, you could think of compost as nothing more than microbe poop. Compost ingredients may include everything from tomato plants to dung to yard clippings. This stuff has been recommended by almost everyone who has anything to do with gardening, from university personnel to your mother. But why?

The practice

Compost is often mixed into the soil prior to planting. Various sources recommend specific quantities of compost for different conditions, but in general 20–30 gallons (about 100 pounds) of moist compost should be applied per 100 square feet. It should be tilled into the soil as deeply as possible before planting. When compost is applied, the amount of fertilizer recommended is usually cut in half. Recently, people involved with organic gardening have started recommending something called compost tea, which is water that has had compost steeped in it. This water is then applied to the soil or even to a plant's foliage. Compost tea is discussed in more detail in chapter 6.

The theory

Compost is organic matter, so it should provide all the benefits of organic matter, including improved water retention, nutrient retention, and drainage, if used properly. Additionally, compost contains all the nutrients that its ingredients accumulated while alive.

The real story

The organic material present in compost is good for the soil, no two ways about it. It improves drainage, water retention, and nutrient availability. Some evidence also indicates that compost will actually inhibit certain nematodes and pathogens (Davidson et al. 2000), including *Fusarium* species (Pharand et al. 2002), which are very dangerous for many plants in vegetable gardens, and *Phytophthora* species, which may cause damage to all kinds of plants (Widmer et al. 1998). Some sources of compost are better than others, and compost that has not been allowed to—well—compost for long enough will actually take up more nutrients than it releases. As a general rule, compost should be at least 6 months old before it is used, but this is dependent upon many factors. Compost always contains some nutrition for plants, but the amount of nutrition depends upon the ingredients used. Compost that includes animal matter, such as fish or feathers, tends to be higher in nitrogen than those composed primarily of vegetable matter. Some types of vegetable matter, such as grapefruit and banana skins, may contain quite a bit of potassium, and other types, such as cantaloupe rinds, may contain a high concentration of phosphorus. None of this nutrition is quickly available to the plant but is instead provided slowly as the components of the compost break down. When compost is added to a garden, enough micronutrients are usually added so that additional micronutrients are not needed.

It is possible that some composts, especially those with a high content of municipal wastes, could include heavy metals. Other contaminants in compost that should be left out if possible include the leaves of certain trees, including walnut and eucalyptus, which may be harmful to the roots of other plants, and the feces of dogs, cats, and humans, as these substances may contain harmful pathogens. The best thing for people with only a small compost requirement is to make it themselves following local extension guides or to purchase it from a reputable company and ask them about heavy metals and biological contaminants in their product.

COMPOST MATERIAL	% N	% P	% K
banana skins (ash)	–	3.25	41.76
cantaloupe rinds (ash)	–	9.77	12.21
castor bean pomace	5.00	2.00	1.00
cattail reeds	2.00	.81	3.43
coffee grounds	2.08	.32	.28
corncob ash	–	–	50.00
corn stalks & leaves	.30	.13	.33
crabgrass, green	.66	.19	.71
eggs, rotten	2.25	.19	.15
feathers	15.30	–	–
fish scrap	2.00–7.50	1.50–6.00	–
grapefruit skins (ash)	–	3.58	30.60
oak leaves	.80	.35	.15
orange culls	.20	.13	.21
pine needles	.46	.12	.03
ragweed	.76	.26	–
tea grounds	4.15	.62	.40
wood ashes	–	1.00	4.0–10.00

Figure 2. The amount of nitrogen, phosphorus, and potassium in organic compost materials as a percentage of dry weight

Source: J. M. Stephens 1994. Courtesy of University of Florida, Institute of Food and Agricultural Sciences

While compost is generally good, always remember that compost is an amendment to soil, and should not be used instead of soil. Growing plants directly in compost does not usually work well.

What it means to you ✿✿✿✿✿

Compost is helpful, but be careful to use good compost in a wise manner. Compost added to a garden will reduce the need for fertilizers and should supply the micronutrients required for normal plant growth.

Eggshells

Eggs are one of nature's great miracles. They contain all that is needed for a tiny creature to emerge, and they also taste good with a little salt and hot sauce. But what could eggshells, the part that's left after the egg has been eaten, possibly do for a garden?

The practice

Eggshells are often recommended as an amendment to soils or media because of their high calcium content. Recommendations tend to be pretty inexact, with anywhere from one to six eggshells recommended for a container. Besides simply adding the eggshells, recommendations may also include boiling them in water and then allowing this mixture to sit for some time, generally 15 minutes to 24 hours, straining out the shells, and using the remaining water to irrigate your plants.

The theory

Eggshells have a high concentration of calcium, which is what gives them their rigidity. If this calcium can get into the soil where the plants are growing, then perhaps it could be taken up and used by the plants.

The real story

Unsurprisingly, when hunting through old literature, I was unable to find any information on what the addition of eggshells might mean for the nutrition of a plant. To address this dilemma I cracked an egg, removed the yolk and white (so as not to be wasteful I made some pancakes), and wiped out the inside so there were no residues left. I then crushed the eggshell into small bits, about the size of aspirin, and boiled them in a few cups of distilled water. After boiling, I let the eggshells sit in the water for 24 hours and then strained them out and collected the water. I sent the eggshell water, along with a sample of the distilled water, to be tested by the University of Minnesota's analytical lab to find out how much extra nutrition the eggshell added to the water. At first this experiment may seem strange because I didn't look at the eggshell in the soil itself, but boiling the eggshell and letting it sit gives a reasonable estimate of the nutrition in the shell that will go into solution and so be quickly available to the plant. Nutrients that did not come out of the eggshell during boiling would probably not be available for the plant to use anytime soon if the eggshells were placed into a soil or media. Additionally, this experiment tells us whether boiling an eggshell in water and saving that water to irrigate plants is a good idea.

Five nutrients were more abundant in the boiled–eggshell water than in the distilled water (although we didn't look at nitrogen, which may have increased also). The first element was sodium. The increase in concentration was relatively small, and it is unlikely that this amount of added sodium would help or hurt the plant. Two other elements that increased were phosphorus and magnesium, but, while these elements are certainly beneficial to plants, their concentrations were very low. Finally, two other elements were released by the eggshell in quantities that might be beneficial to a plant. About 4 milligrams of both calcium and potassium were released into the water. Okay, okay. Four milligrams is really small, but if you were to boil, say, ten or twenty eggshells (a realistic number to produce during a hard day of baking) in a gallon of water, you would have a nice little calcium and potassium amendment to add to your soil or media.

Before closing this section, I have to admit that I should have tested 10 or 20 eggshells from 10 or 20 different sources and then tested chicken eggshells against the eggshells of different bird, or even reptile, species. Hopefully someone else out there will run these tests and publish his or her results. Every new experiment lends a little more to our understanding of the world around us.

What it means to you ❀❀❀❀❀

Eggshells shouldn't be your only source of fertilizer, but eggshells are a waste product that we typically throw away without thinking twice. Why not use them to provide added nutrition for your plants? Based on the results I found—and my results were, again, based on only one test—I would use four or five eggshells per plant, mixed into the soil in a garden situation, and the same number mixed into the media prior to planting in containers. Additionally, boiling ten to twenty eggshells in a gallon of water for a few minutes (watch out though—I found out the hard way that this mix tends to bubble over), letting the mix sit overnight, and straining the eggshells ought to provide a nice amendment to apply once every week or two. Or if it's more convenient, you could just take the water you use to make hardboiled eggs and apply this to the soil or medium that your plants are in. Two cups of this solution per plant ought to be appropriate. I would not store the concoction for longer than a day. Though I haven't tested it, I would be surprised if the water used for boiling other foods, such as vegetables, isn't also beneficial for feeding plants.

Epsom salts 🌱

Epsom salts are sold in garden centers as a classic concoction to add to many fertilizer homebrews, but few people really know what Epsom salts are. Are you dying to know the answer? Okay, here it is. Epsom salts are a simple salt composed of two nutrients, magnesium and sulfur, as can easily be discerned by the chemical formula $MgSO_4$. Epsom salts are so named because they were first collected from mineral springs in Epsom, England. These salts can benefit our gardens, but not always in ways the gurus would have us believe.

The practice

Epsom salts are often dissolved in water and applied as a liquid fertilizer, either to the soil or as a foliar spray. The concentration used for this type of application is usually about ¼ cup of these salts for every gallon of water, which should cover 1000 square feet. Epsom salts can also be applied dry to the surface of the soil. In this case ¼–½ cup of Epsom salts is applied around the base of the plant.

The theory

Epsom salts contain two elements critical to plant growth, magnesium and sulfur. Proponents of this classic concoction adhere to the theory that plants are often deficient in these two elements. Some people also think Epsom salts decrease pH.

The real story

There is no doubt that some plants, such as poinsettias, chrysanthemums, kalanchoes, and gardenias, often have high levels of magnesium in their leaves (Dole and Wilkins 1999; Mills and Jones 1996). Therefore, they may benefit from higher levels of this element in their soil or media. Most planting media contain sufficient magnesium for normal growth, though, and adding Epsom salts is unnecessary for most plants in most situations.

Where magnesium is deficient, the soil is likely to be acidic. In these conditions it is more appropriate to add dolomitic lime rather than Epsom salts because dolomitic lime will increase pH as well as add magnesium. If soil is at an appropriate pH already, then Epsom salts are the better addition (Jokinen 1982).

Although Epsom salts have been reported to make soils more acidic, there is little evidence to indicate this. Epsom salts are considered neutral salts, meaning they will have little effect on the pH of soil or media.

What it means to you ❀❀❀❀

Epsom salts are a handy way to deliver two nutrients, sulfur and magnesium, to a plant, and if your plant is low in either of these, there is a benefit to adding this salt. Epsom salts are not magic and don't take the place of other nutrients. Epsom salts are not generally harmful to add to your plants, but they are usually unnecessary. In many, if not most, cases where there is little magnesium in the soil, there is also an acid pH. In these cases dolomitic lime is more appropriate than Epsom salts as a way to add magnesium.

It would be convenient if I could provide an easy way to tell whether your plant needs magnesium or sulfur, but I can't. If you are seeing a nutrient deficiency, it is best to have your soil tested to find out why the deficiency is occurring. This is usually best done through your state extension service. By applying something, such as Epsom salts, without testing your soil, you are simply rolling the dice to find the cure. You may be right, but you may make things worse.

Gypsum 🌱

Gypsum is touted as the way to make your garden soil alive again. In fact Edmund Ruffin (1832) once wrote, "There is no operation of nature less understood . . . as the enormous increase of vegetable growth from a very small quantity of gypsum, *in circumstances favourable to its action*" (my emphasis). This soil amendment is often referred to as a soil "loosener," but, as with Epsom salts, few people really understand exactly what gypsum is and what it is supposed to do. Let's make it easy. Gypsum is calcium sulfate, which basically offers two nutrients: calcium and sulfur. Can adding these nutrients in the form of gypsum improve your soil?

The practice

Gypsum is applied at various concentrations and is usually incorporated into the soil prior to planting. I have seen recommendations to apply as much as 6 pounds of gypsum per 100 square feet.

The theory

Gypsum is supposed to loosen soils, making them easier to work and allowing air and water to more easily reach the root system of plants, thereby effectively revitalizing the soil. It supposedly accomplishes this by displacing sodium ions in the soil.

The real story

Gypsum does indeed displace sodium ions in the soil when it is applied where high amounts of sodium are present, such as occurs in soils in the western United States and in coastal areas (Bauder and Brock 2001; Alam et al. 2002). The displacement of sodium gives the soil much better structure. Additionally, gypsum supplies calcium and sulfur. If these elements are lacking in a planting medium, gypsum is a good amendment.

Because gypsum is a neutral salt, it is especially valuable when you want to increase soil calcium without raising pH. Typically, lime is used to provide calcium, but when you want to avoid increasing the alkalinity of a soil, gypsum is the perfect amendment. Gypsum's main drawback is that people often think it is a good soil additive under most conditions. While gypsum is rarely harmful when applied following the label instructions, it will only benefit soils and media under certain conditions. Additional claims are usually unfounded.

What it means to you ❀❀❀❀

Under high-sodium soil conditions, gypsum is a very valuable amendment. It is especially useful in certain parts of the United States, mostly in the West and in coastal areas, where sodium builds up in soils and makes them crusty, badly affecting a plant's ability to grow and thrive. Gypsum is also valuable in conditions where a soil needs calcium or sulfur but where pH is already close to optimal. I always use gypsum when planting tomatoes in containers on my back porch, as these vegetables have a relatively high demand for calcium but usually don't need to have the pH of their media altered. Gypsum is, like Epsom salts, not usually harmful to add to a soil, but it is not needed nearly as often as people think. As with Epsom salts, the best way to find out if you need gypsum is to have your soil tested.

Lime ☙

Lime has been used in agriculture since Roman times, when Lucius Junius Moderatus Columella wrote about his uncle, Marcus Columella, who used chalk or marl (basically a naturally occurring calcium deposit) to improve gravelly soils (Columella 1745).

Lime is usually composed primarily of calcium carbonate, though other compounds may also be present. A number of different types of lime are sold, but the most common ones found in garden centers are hydrated lime (calcium hydroxide) and dolomitic lime. These two types have different characteristics, so that care needs to be taken when choosing one.

The practice

Lime is usually purchased as a powder and spread across an area that is too acidic to grow healthy plants. It can be either incorporated into the soil or placed on top of it to increase pH. Recommendations for lime vary from 1 to 5 pounds of lime per 100 square feet, depending upon the type of lime used and the amount of pH change desired.

The theory

After application, the chemicals in lime undergo a reaction that causes the soil or medium to become more alkaline (have a higher pH). This should be beneficial to plants in situations where the soil or medium is too acidic for optimal growth. Additionally, lime adds calcium and magnesium to soils.

The real story

Although lime has long been known to have potential benefits for soils, the reason for these benefits was unknown until Edmund Ruffin, better known for claiming to have fired the first shot in the American Civil War and committing suicide at its conclusion because he could not stand the "vile Yankee race," published a book titled *An Essay on Calcareous Manures* (1832). His book related how lime could affect a soil's chemistry by making it more alkaline, something he established after reading Humphry Davy's book *Elements of Agricultural Chemistry* (1814), which included information on experiments conducted around 1755 by a Dr. Black in Edinburgh. Those experiments demonstrated that limestone and chalk become alkaline when heated.

The two different types of lime commonly used in gardens, hydrated lime and dolomitic lime, have different properties and affect the soil differently. Hydrated lime tends to react very quickly with the soil and rapidly alters pH. Because it reacts so quickly, it unfortunately also dissipates quickly and does not provide a lasting effect on pH. Dolomitic lime reacts more slowly than hydrated lime and is less water soluble, which provides a more lasting effect on pH. Additionally, dolomitic lime usually contains more magnesium than hydrated lime. To complicate matters just a little bit more, the size of the lime particles will also affect how quickly it works and how effective it is at altering pH. Larger particles react more slowly, and smaller particles react more rapidly.

Lime definitely helps plants in situations where soil pH may be too low (too acidic) for plants to grow normally. Lime will also increase the amount of calcium and magnesium plants have available to them (Wright et al. 1999). Phosphorus, potassium, sulfur, calcium, and magnesium are all more available to plants at a higher pH. However, if the lime pushes pH too high, then other elements, such as zinc, manganese, and especially iron, will not be as available to your plants. Containers often include media that are very acidic; in situations where this is the case, lime is beneficial to plant growth, but be careful because too much lime will result in reduced growth (Gillman et al. 1998). If pH is already at an appropriate level, lime can even damage plants. As far back as the 1890s lime was known to injure certain plants, including conifers, rhododendrons, and azaleas (Henderson 1890).

People who have been farming for a long time say lime sweetens the soil. I'm not exactly sure what "sweetening the soil" is—it is certainly not a commonly used term today—but I suspect it means that nutrients are made more available to the plant because of lime additions. If this is indeed what it means, then lime sweetens the soil only when the natural pH is too low.

What it means to you ❋❋❋❋

If pH is too low in your soil or medium, adding some form of lime will definitely help. Lime will also help with calcium and magnesium if these elements are lacking in the soil, but it should not be added if calcium or magnesium deficiency are the only problems. Epsom salts and gypsum are more appropriate in these situations because they do not alter soil or media pH the way that lime will. The amount of lime to add to a particular site is extremely variable and depends on the type of soil, type of lime, and environmental conditions you have in your area. Contact your local extension service or talk to a knowledgeable garden center employee to get recommendations. Lime can have lasting deleterious effects on a lawn or garden if it is not used properly.

Liquid, granular, and slow-release fertilizers

What type of fertilizer should you buy? There are all kinds of options; you can buy liquid, granular, or slow-release fertilizers. But is there a difference between them? Should we care whether we use a liquid rather than a slow-release fertilizer?

The practice

Fertilizer is nothing more than various types of nutritional salts mixed together. These salts can be delivered to a soil or medium in a solid form, typically called granular fertilizer, or mixed in water, typically called liquid fertilizer (you can also buy this as a powder to mix with water yourself).

There is also something called slow-release fertilizer, which is basically a granular fertilizer that has been covered with some kind of coating, usually plastic, so that it will release its nutrients more slowly.

The theory

Theoretically, the three different fertilizers are useful in different situations. Liquid fertilizers should be more useful for plants that need a quick shot of nutrition or for situations where fertilizer will be applied multiple times throughout a growing season. Slow-release fertilizers are supposed to be best for plants that need a constant stream of fertilizer and for situations where you just don't have enough time to continuously reapply fertilizer. Granular fertilizers are primarily for outdoor situations, where cost and labor are concerns, as these fertilizers are usually among the cheapest, and easiest, to apply.

The real story

The major difference among the fertilizer delivery systems is the rate at which the salts dissolve and deliver nutrition to the plants. This difference matters more in certain situations. In containers, for example, nutrients move through media rapidly. Multiple applications of a fertilizer that dissolves rapidly, or fewer applications of a fertilizer that dissolves slowly, are required. On soil, however, nutrients tend to hang around, allowing the plant to use them for a longer period of time; in soil, even highly soluble fertilizers will be available to the plant for at least a few weeks. Clay soils tend to hold nutrients for a longer period of time than sandy soils.

The various types of fertilizer all have their merits, and all deliver nutrients to the plant. Some methods, however, are more effective than others in particular situations. Liquid fertilizers are sold as salts either already dissolved in water or that will easily dissolve in water. Because of their solubility, these salts move quickly through the soil with rain or any sort of irrigation and need to be applied quite frequently. The rapid movement enables them to reach the plants' roots quickly, but they are also rapidly lost. This delivery system is commonly used in the container production of floriculture crops because of the control that the producer has over the concentration of nutrients. In the home, these fertilizers are useful early in the spring to encourage new growth. When the plant has grown large enough and you want to encourage blooms, liquid fertilization can be stopped, and the fertilizer will flush out of the media relatively rapidly.

Granular fertilizers are usually the cheapest. The salts that make up these products are typically not as soluble as those that make up liquid fertilizers, so their nutrients tend to last for a longer period of time than those delivered as a liquid. These fertilizers are preferred when large areas need to be covered. Simply because of cost, this delivery system is the one most commonly used for lawns and in the care and production of trees grown in the ground.

Slow-release fertilizers are granular fertilizers that have been coated with some material, usually plastic, that allows nutrients to be delivered more slowly than either of the other fertilizer delivery methods. This type of fertilization is most commonly used in containers because containers cannot hold large amounts of nutrients for long periods of time. Slow-release fertilizers are used for the production of trees and shrubs in containers and is also very convenient for home fertilization. The release of nutrients from slow-release fertilizers depends on the type you buy, how often and how much your plants are watered, and temperature. The higher the temperature and the more water applied, the less time they will last.

What it means to you ❀❀❀❀

There are distinct benefits to each type of fertilizer delivery system. For plants living in containers or for anyplace where we want to see rapid growth and will have the opportunity to reapply often, liquid fertilizer is a good option. In large areas, such as lawns and gardens, granular fertilizers make sense because they are economical and will last for a reasonably long time in the soil. Slow-release fertilizers are the most expensive form and are most appropriately used for plants growing in containers, where you do not want to be bothered with reapplying fertilizer often. Slow-release fertilizers are also a good idea in gardens with sandy soils, where other fertilizers might leach through too quickly.

Micronutrient mixes

Micronutrient mixes are commercial formulations of the micronutrients that plants need but that are not present in many of the synthetic fertilizers. These mixes include many elements that plants need in small quantities, such as boron, copper, manganese, molybdenum, and zinc. We are told that we need these products to ensure that we have good plants. Is this true?

The practice

Micronutrient mixes are usually applied as a spray to a plant's foliage or as a granular application to soil or media. These products typically contain many elements that are needed for plant growth but are not needed in the same quantity as the macronutrients (nitrogen, phosphorus, potassium, calcium, magnesium, and sulfur). Micronutrients are applied at very low concentrations and are sometimes even incorporated into regular liquid, granular, and slow-release fertilizers, in which case additional applications of micronutrient mixes would rarely be necessary.

The theory

It is well established that plants need micronutrients; the theory is that micronutrient mixes will supply these necessary elements and alleviate any possible nutrient deficiency.

The real story

Sixteen elements are essential to plant growth: boron, calcium, carbon, chlorine, copper, hydrogen, iron, magnesium, manganese, molybdenum, nitrogen, oxygen, phosphorus, potassium, sulfur, and zinc. Scientists learned that these elements are essential by attempting to grow plants without them. They found that without these elements plants will not grow and will eventually die. Micronutrient mixes aim to prevent nutrient deficiency in your soil or media by offering elements that could be lacking and are not supplied by typical synthetic fertilizers. Organic fertilizers are different from synthetics because they generally include more micronutrients, and when organic fertilizers are properly used, extra micronutrients are rarely needed. Compost will also supply micronutrients to plants.

Since we know micronutrients are necessary for plant growth, it is just common sense that an application of a micronutrient fertilizer will help supply any missing micronutrients. Plants growing in containers are more likely to be in a micronutrient-deficient situation than plants growing in good soil, especially when the media are composed primarily of pine bark (Wright et al. 1999).

Many people who use micronutrient mixes assume that just because they are applying micronutrients, they are solving their micronutrient problems, but this is not always the case. Often there is a problem in the soil, such as a very low or high pH, that will make a particular nutrient unavailable to the plant no matter how much of it is added (Mengel and Kirkby 1987). In these situations a chelate can be added to correct nutrient problems.

What it means to you ❋❋❋

Micronutrient mixes work if your planting medium is lacking in these nutrients; the mixes are certainly worth a try if you feel you have been experiencing less-than-optimal growth from your plants. This is especially true when your plants are growing in containers. The reason micronutrients don't receive four or five points is that most soils do contain enough micronutrients for the plants that people are trying to grow. However, if a soil or medium is devoid of some micronutrient, these products may prove incredibly useful. For people who use organic fertilizers or compost, an application of micronutrients is often a waste of money. If you decide that a micronutrient mix is right for you, make sure you have checked the pH of your soil before expecting benefits; a pH that is too high or too low will lead to micronutrient deficiencies no matter how much micronutrient mix is added.

Organic fertilizers 🌱

Organic fertilizers—such as bone meal, dried blood, fish emulsion fertilizers, guano, manure, and others—are simply fertilizers that have been derived from a natural source. Because they come from a natural source, they are assumed to be earth friendly and possibly better for a plant than synthetic fertilizers. It should come as no surprise that organic fertilizers have been around for a lot longer than synthetic fertilizers. In Roman times a number of different types of dung were used, with pigeon dung considered the best (Columella 1745). By the late 1800s dung was still the standard, but more types of dung were being utilized. Commercial fertilizers utilizing Peruvian guano (bat guano) and bone dust headed the list of those most commonly used. During that time, fertilizers made of mixtures of different types of dung and other natural products became popular, perhaps because of the differing concentrations of nutrients in the various products. One of those fertilizers was comprised of guano or bone dust, leaf mould, well pulverized dry muck, sweepings from a paved street, and rotted stable manure (Henderson 1890). Finding old nuggets of information like this one makes my job interesting.

The practice

Gardeners who want to use only natural products on their land will frequently use fertilizers that are advertised as "organic," such as bone meal, various forms of guano, and fish products. These fertilizers are usually applied to the soil, but some, such as fish emulsions, may be applied to foliage.

The theory

Organic fertilizers should supply nutrition to a plant in the same way synthetic fertilizers do, but at a lower dose. Organic fertilizers are also supposed to offer more nutrients and release them more slowly than synthetic fertilizers.

The real story

Organic fertilizers generally have a much lower analysis of nutrients than synthetic fertilizers do. (Also see the entry "Analyzing the ever-changing fertilizer analysis".) In other words, organic fertilizers generally include a smaller percentage of nitrogen, phosphorus, and potassium than synthetic fertilizers. A fertilizer made of fish scraps may have an analysis as low as 5-3-0. The low analyses mean that more of these fertilizers must be applied to a particular soil or container to get the same effect as a smaller amount of synthetic fertilizer.

Fertilizers that are organic have the advantage of releasing nutrients more slowly than those that are liquid or granular. (Also see the entry "Liquid, granular, and slow-release fertilizers".) The release is slower because the nutrients are chemically bonded to organic compounds (hence the name "organic fertilizers"). As the nutrients separate from the organic compounds over time, they become available for the plant to use. Because these fertilizers release nutrients more slowly, they need to be applied less often than most synthetic fertilizers, with the exception of slow-release fertilizers.

Organic fertilizers also tend to affect the pH of a soil with repeated use. Different organic fertilizers will have different pH effects, and if you are using a single type of organic fertilizer repeatedly you should be aware of its probable effects on the pH of your soil.

I have heard garden gurus suggest that organic fertilizers cannot burn plants like synthetic fertilizers can. Having burned plants with organic fertilizer myself, I can reliably say the gurus are wrong. Fertilizer burn occurs

ORGANIC MATERIALS	% N	% P	% K	AVAILABILITY	ACIDITY
fish scrap	5.0	3.0	0	slowly	acid
fish meal	10.0	4.0	0	slowly	acid
guano, Peru	13.0	8.0	2.0	moderately	acid
guano, bat	10.0	4.0	2.0	moderately	acid
sewage sludge	2.0-6.0	1.0-2.5	0.0-0.4	slowly	acid
dried blood	12.0	1.5	0.8	moderately slow	acid
soybean meal	7.0	1.2	1.5	slowly	very slightly acid
tankage, animal	9.0	10.0	15.5	slowly	acid
tankage, garbage	2.5	1.5	1.5	very slowly	alkaline
tobacco stems	1.5	0.5	5.0	slowly	alkaline
seaweed	1.0	–	4.0-10.0	slowly	–
bone meal, raw	3.5	22.0	–	slowly	alkaline
urea	45.0	–	–	quickly	acid
castor pomace	6.0	1.2	0.5	slowly	acid
wood ashes	–	2.0	4.0-10.0	quickly	alkaline
cocoa shell meal	2.5	1.0	2.5	slowly	neutral
cotton seed meal	6.0	2.5	1.5	slowly	acid
ground rock phosphate	–	33.0	–	very slowly	alkaline
green sand	–	1.0	6.0	very slowly	–
basic slag	–	8.0	–	quickly	alkaline
horn and hoof meal	12.0	2.0	–	–	–
milorganite	6.0	2.5	–	–	–
peat and muck	1.5-3.0	0.25-0.5	0.5-.10	very slowly	acid
spent mushroom compost	2.0	0.74	1.46	moderately	6.4

Figure 3. The dry-weight percentage and availability of nitrogen, phosphorus, and potassium in typical organic fertilizers, as well their effects on pH

Source: J. M. Stephens 1994. Courtesy of University of Florida, Institute of Food and Agricultural Sciences

when something high in salt, such as fertilizer, is placed next to growing plant tissue. The salt will cause the plant's cells to desiccate (because of the osmotic potential created by the salt), leading to cell death and a burned look. Fertilizer burn can be avoided by applying the proper amount of fertilizer to your yard or garden—using recommendations on the fertilizer label or from your state extension service—and by making sure your plant is well watered. Organic fertilizers usually do contain a lower concentration of salts than synthetic fertilizers and are therefore less likely to burn plants, but it is far from impossible.

A second, lesser-known problem with organic fertilizers concerns ammonia. Ammonia is released from fresh manure at a concentration that is damaging to plants, so it is best to compost manure for at least 6 months before using it.

Contrary to common belief, there is no evidence organic fertilizers have any benefit beyond the basic nutrients they deliver. They do come from previously living things and therefore do contain micronutrients that may be valuable to plant growth, but besides these there really isn't anything that would make organic fertilizers behave any differently from synthetic fertilizers. If misapplied, they could still pollute the environment or hurt your plants.

What it means to you ❀❀❀❀❀

Organic fertilizers earn a score of five for a few reasons. First, although they are generally more expensive than synthetic fertilizers, they supply additional micronutrients that many synthetic fertilizers do not, and they last longer. Additionally, organic fertilizers are a renewable resource. Remember, though, that there is no magic behind them; they deliver nutrients to the plant the same as any synthetic fertilizer does. They are very useful, but despite being organic, they can still cause fertilizer burn and pollution just as synthetic fertilizers can.

Shampoo and liquid soaps

Many of the home-brewed helpers that garden gurus recommend include soaps. These soaps usually come in the form of either shampoo (typically baby shampoo) or some other type of liquid soap. Most people don't have a clue as to what these products are supposed to do.

The practice

Suggestions commonly range from 1 to 2 tablespoons to 1 cup of some type of shampoo or liquid soap added to other ingredients, usually ammonia or beer, for a fertilizer. This concoction is then sprayed on the garden with a hose-end sprayer.

The theory

According to theory, applying shampoos and soaps will help to soften soils. Unfortunately "soft soil" is not a well-understood phrase, and it is difficult to qualify exactly what it means. The phrase is usually used to indicate the amount of organic matter in the soil, with softer soils having higher concentrations of organic matter. However, it is sometimes also used to indicate a soil with a low salt content or that is easily wet.

The real story

To properly investigate what soap may do to the soil we should first look at the three things garden gurus may mean when they refer to soap as a soil softener. First, soap will not add any organic matter to the soil, so this (hopefully!) is not what the gurus are referring to. Next, if a soil is high in salt there is little reason to believe that an application of soap will do anything that regular water wouldn't, so, again, this is probably not what the garden gurus mean. What about helping the soil to get wet? Well, here the gurus may have something. Soaps may act as so-called wetting agents, which allow water to move through soil more quickly and more easily, especially soils that are normally resistant to water moving through them, and may increase the amount of water the soil holds. The actual practice of adding wetting agents to improve plant health and growth, however, has met with mixed results. In a study in New Zealand that looked at sandy soils, wetting agents seemed to be generally beneficial (Wallis et al. 1990), but in another study that looked at how soaps increased yield in potatoes, very little benefit was realized (Lowery et al. 2004). The best way to summarize the potential benefits of wetting agents is simply to say that, depending on the conditions you have in your garden, they may be helpful. Unfortunately, it is difficult to pinpoint exactly what those conditions are.

Wetting agents are a tried-and-true practice in one situation. Commercially produced wetting agents are extremely useful for container media because these media often have peat in them. Peat that has been allowed to dry, such as what you find on most garden center shelves, is notoriously difficult to wet; wetting agents are useful for keeping these media watered (Nelson 2003). Wetting agents could be especially helpful in situations where plants are being grown in containers and water conservation is a concern, as you can probably get by with less water per watering when wetting agents are added to media (Bilderback et al. 1997).

What it means to you 🏵🏵

Because most of the plants you buy in containers already contain wetting agents, there is little reason to believe that soap will benefit them, and it may even hurt since soaps have a tendency to burn leaves if misapplied. Adding soap to soils to increase water infiltration may work if the soil is resistant to watering, but since most soils, and especially well-tilled garden soils, are not resistant to watering, adding these soaps is largely a waste of time. Besides, it is always a questionable practice to add things to a soil that were never intended to be there, like shampoo. Commercial wetting agents have been created specifically for soils; shampoo has been created specifically for hair and should not be expected to be an effective soil softener. Furthermore, a long, deep watering of the ground is likely to be just as effective at getting water to the roots of your plants as applying a liquid soap or shampoo, if not more effective.

Soda, syrup, and other sugary snacks

Sugary substances are often recommended as plant fertilizers. I have seen soda, syrup, molasses, and even sugar suggested as a pick-me-up for gardens. Will these sugary snacks rot plant life the same way they rot your teeth, or are they just the thing to cure an ailing plant?

The practice

Sugar is usually applied to the garden in combination with a few other components. Common homemade fertilizer recipes include a cup or so of beer, a can of soda, a little soap (between a tablespoon and a cup), and some ammonia. This concoction is then applied with a hose-end sprayer onto the area to be fertilized. Other recipes may include from 3 to 10 ounces of sugar dissolved in a gallon of water to be applied at the time of transplant.

The theory

All these sugary things contain one common ingredient, sugar, in one form or another. Most of the proponents for feeding sugary substances to plants believe that these substances feed good bacteria in the soil, but some think the sugar may serve as a food, or even a root stimulant, for the plant.

The real story

To elucidate the effects of some of my favorite sugar sources—cola, lemon-lime soda, molasses, and syrup—on plant health, I ran a little test of their effects on plants. This test used hydroponics, just like the test of beer. To 5½ gallons of water, we added either 6 or 12 ounces of cola, 6 or 12 ounces of a lemon-lime soda, 1 or 2 tablespoons of molasses, or 2 tablespoons of syrup. The water contained a low level of nutrition, as in the tests with beer (enough nutrition to keep the plants alive, but not enough to really get them growing). After about 2 days, the plants had a tremendous increase in bacteria growing on their roots. Just like in the beer tests, this bacteria didn't help the growth of the plants. Interestingly, both molasses treatments fared better than the other treatments. Those of you who were hoping the molasses might provide astounding growth will be disappointed to note that the plants that received no sugar at all still performed the best.

So has anyone actually looked at what sugar might do to a plant growing in a landscape rather than in a bucket of water? Yes, someone has. A paper published in 2005 by two Englishmen, Glynn Percival and Gillian Fraser, looked at various types of sugars, including fructose, galactose, glucose, maltose, rhamnose, and sucrose, to see whether the addition of any of these sugars to irrigation water at the time of transplanting (a time when the root system is greatly reduced) would benefit birch trees. Two of these sugars, fructose and glucose, are commonly found in soft drinks and other sweet treats, so this study offers some insight into whether tooth-rotting beverages and treats could benefit young trees.

The researchers found that some of the sugars—fructose, glucose, and sucrose—did speed up the root development of birch trees when applied at a concentration of anywhere from 3 to 10 ounces of sugar per gallon of water once a week for 4 weeks after transplanting. Just under a half gallon (1.5 liters) of the sugar solution was applied per irrigation, and no other irrigation source was offered. This research is very interesting and certainly opens the door to the possibility that sugary snacks might benefit plants; unfortunately, these treatments also had some negative effects, such as apparently decreasing photosynthesis. The findings are enough to lead me to think that sugar might be beneficial to tree growth in situations where a tree's root system is highly compromised, but they are far from conclusive because only one type of tree was examined and because there is a lack of other research supporting the conclusions of this paper. But who knows? It is well within the realm of possibility that some other researcher will give sugar a shot and will find results that support the idea of feeding it to plants at the time of transplanting, in which case you can be sure that I'll amend this book.

You should consider both experiments when determining whether a sugary snack is right for your plants. Applying sugar will increase bacteria, which may have a negative effect on your plants, but there is evidence that when a plant's root system has been highly compromised, such as during transplanting, a few applications of sugar may help to stimulate root development, at least in birch trees.

What it means to you ❀❀

Weird sources of sugar should not be considered a good way to encourage growth under normal growing conditions; they are likely to increase bacterial growth that could be hazardous to roots. However, in a situation where the roots of a tree or shrub have been cut, there is evidence, though far from conclusive, that sugar might help to encourage root development. Perhaps you might wonder whether I would apply sugar to my own newly planted Japanese maple (or ash, or oak, or crabapple). Not a chance, at least not until more research is conducted.

Sulfur, iron sulfate, aluminum sulfate, and other soil acidifiers ☙

These compounds are intended to lower the pH of soils or media that are too alkaline for a plant. They are similar to chelates in that both are intended for plants that have been placed in a site that is too alkaline for them.

Even back in the 1870s one of these compounds, iron sulfate, was noted as a good way to deliver iron to pear trees (William 1871a). It probably achieved this more through acidifying the soil (allowing iron already in the soil to reach the plant) than through the actual iron it delivered.

The practice

Sulfur, iron sulfate, and aluminum sulfate are applied to soils at various concentrations to reduce pH. Other soil acidifiers are applied at different concentrations depending on their ingredients, which might include ammonium sulfate, urea, a variety of acids, or other chemicals.

The theory

Soil acidifiers are supposed to react chemically with the soil to produce acidic conditions. Addition of soil acidifiers that are themselves acidic, such as phosphoric acid, should cause a soil to become even more acidic.

The real story

Soil acidifiers may contain a variety of active compounds. These compounds do acidify the soil and will result in increased uptake of nutrients that are more available in acid conditions; iron and manganese are the two elements most commonly unavailable to plants due to alkaline soils. Other compounds that help acidify the soil, including ammonium sulfate, urea, and others, also contain a certain amount of nutrition and can deliver nutrients at the same time that pH is being altered.

If pH adjustment is all you want to accomplish, and you are not interested in adding fertilizer, then the best choices for acidifying your soil or media include sulfur, aluminum sulfate, and iron sulfate. Sulfur tends to act

MATERIAL	SANDY LOAM	LOAM	CLAY LOAM OR PEAT
aluminum sulfate	2.5	5	7
iron sulfate	2.5	5	7
sulfur	0.5	1	1.5

Figure 4. The number of pounds of aluminum sulfate, iron sulfate, and sulfur needed per 100 square feet to decrease pH by one level in various soil types. These amendments are most effective when incorporated into the soil.

Source: Swanson et al. 1986. Reviewed on June 1, 2005

slowly in the soil, and it may take a long time for this element to drop the pH to a level that is appropriate for the plants you want to grow. Sulfur is also relatively insoluble, so it will not move through the soil profile too rapidly. That means it will provide pH control for a long period of time, perhaps even 3 or 4 years, depending on soil conditions. Iron and aluminum sulfate have the advantage of altering pH more quickly than plain sulfur, but because they are more soluble they tend to flow through a medium and offer much less in the way of long-term pH control. In sandier soils only about a year of pH control should be expected. Acids added to soils to change pH are usually quite soluble and will only provide short-term pH correction.

What it means to you ❀❀❀❀

Sulfur, iron sulfate, aluminum sulfate, and other soil acidifiers will accomplish what they say they will, but sulfur is cheaper and will offer a longer-term pH control than any other option. If you do decide to use sulfur, try to incorporate it into your soil, as it will not penetrate the earth rapidly on its own. For plants that are in soils much too alkaline, a rapid pH change may be in order. In this case iron or aluminum sulfate will work well, as will any soil acidifier applied at the proper concentration. Be careful when using iron or aluminum sulfate. These compounds are stronger salts than sulfur, meaning that an overapplication can be quite dangerous for your garden. Aluminum can be toxic to your plants, so you need to be especially careful not to overapply aluminum sulfate.

Vinegar

Vinegar is recommended as a soil or media amendment for many different plants that like acidic conditions, such as azaleas, camellias, and blueberries. It can also be used as a fungicide or herbicide; those uses are discussed in chapters 6 and 7.

The practice

The common recommendation is for about 2 tablespoons of vinegar in 1 quart of water. It is recommended that this recipe be added to the media of potted plants or to the soil of outdoor plants. This recipe is most often recommended for azalea.

The theory

Vinegar is acidic; therefore if added to a soil it should acidify the soil, allowing plants that prefer acid conditions to thrive. This theory is very similar to the one behind using commercially produced acids to alter pH.

The real story

Since vinegar is acidic, there is no doubt that it will acidify the soil, at least to some extent. Because vinegar mixes well with water, it will not be able to keep the pH of the soil or media low for very long and will rapidly wash through the container or soil profile. This differentiates vinegar from commercial soil acidifiers that are based on acids: commercial acidifiers don't move through the soil as rapidly. In fact, I found that adding apple cider vinegar to containers at a concentration of 2 tablespoons per 1 quart of water did not lower the pH of the medium in the container for longer than a single watering, but my results will not hold true for all vinegars because they differ in their acidity.

What it means to you ❀❀

I would not use my pricy bottle of balsamic vinegar on azaleas. The effects wouldn't last nearly as long as commercial acidifiers, such as sulfur or iron sulfate, and I would mourn the needless loss of the one thing that makes iceberg lettuce worth eating. Nonetheless, for people who want to try out this home-brewed remedy, I can think of worse things to apply. If you do decide to try vinegar, I strongly recommend sticking with one type once you find one that works. You will also need to experiment to determine how often to apply the vinegar. Remember that organic gardeners also use vinegar as an herbicide and that adding too much could be quite bad for your plants. If I were to use vinegar I certainly would not add it every day; once a week is a good place to start.

Putting it all together

From the number of products and recipes listed in this chapter, you might get the idea that it's quite difficult to fertilize a garden. That's not really the case. Yes, you need to be conscientious and thoughtful in order to do it right, but your brain won't melt from mental gyrations trying to figure out the fertilizers and amendments that are best for your situation.

Should you add an amendment?

Most soils, except those extremely high in organic matter (over 10 percent—many soil labs include this information in a normal soil test), can use an amendment of compost. It will help your soil in a variety of ways, including improved water relations, increased nutrient availability, and perhaps even improved soil pH.

Compost is best when it comes from a variety of different sources, such as eggs, fish waste, and banana peels, because different sources contain higher concentrations of different nutrients. As a gardener, you want to add all the nutrients your plants will need. By regularly adding good-quality compost to your garden, you will rarely have to add micronutrients from a micronutrient mix or from an organic fertilizer.

To make sure you are adding nutrients instead of sucking up nutrients when applying compost, it is a good idea to use compost that is at least 6 months old. An easy way to judge whether or not materials have been composting long enough is to take a close look at your compost pile and see if you can recognize the items that went into it. If you can, you probably want to wait a little longer. About 100 pounds of compost per 100 square feet, tilled as deeply into the soil as possible, is the best way to go. If you don't have 100 pounds available, adding whatever you can is better than adding nothing at all. Compost can be added to a soil yearly, and it should be added at least once every 3 or 4 years. I like to make additions during the spring or fall because that is when we till up the garden anyway.

Adding compost to your soil is certainly beneficial, but it isn't a cureall. In any fertility program, it is important to take a soil test to establish the pH of your soil and to find out if any important nutrients are lacking. These tests can be conducted yearly, but usually every 3 or 4 years is sufficient. Testing the soil is often best done a few days after adding compost so that its benefits will be taken into account.

Once you know your soil pH, it's time to look at the preferences of the plants you want to grow. Appendix 1 lists the preferred pH of many different plants. If you cannot find the plant you are working with in the appendix, you may try other sources, such as the store where you bought the plant, but if no recommendations can be found you are usually (but not always!) pretty safe in assuming the plant will perform satisfactorily in a pH of 5.5–6.5. If your ground is not at, or close to, this range, it is best to use a soil acidifier to lower the pH or lime to increase it. These products should be incorporated into the soil with tilling if possible, but if you already have plants in the area, you will need to apply these products to the top of the soil. If you do this, try not to let these products touch stems or roots, as they could injure the plant (though not usually fatally). The entry "Sulfur, iron sulfate, aluminum sulfate, and other soil acidifiers" gives guidelines about adding acidifiers to various types of soil. For lime it is best to check with local experts, preferably from your state extension service, to get recommendations. Those of you who hate to ask for recommendations are relatively safe adding 4 pounds of dolomitic lime per 100 square feet (a 10 foot by 10 foot piece of ground) per year to most acid soils, but for some soils this quantity will be either ineffective or too much. Again, it is best to check with a local expert.

Other amendments that might be important to you at the time of planting include gypsum and Epsom salts. Gypsum is more likely to be beneficial than Epsom salts, especially in coastal areas where salt concentrations may be high, but only a soil test can really tell you what you need. Some people actually taste soil to see whether it is salty or not. If the soil tastes salty, they take it as an indication to apply gypsum. I prefer a soil test.

How should you fertilize?

When your soil is the right pH and all the amendments you need or want are added, it is time to worry about fertilizer. Some people like to incorporate fertilizer into the soil or media at planting, but I don't. If a chunk of fertilizer comes into contact with a plant's roots, it can negatively affect the growth of the plant. I prefer to wait 1 or 2 weeks for annuals and perennials and a few months to a year for trees before I fertilize. Fertilization is a little different for grass, where nutrients are usually added at the time of planting and again later in the year. But how much fertilizer to use? Most fertilizers include instructions on how much should be added to particular crops to achieve the results you want. In general these instructions are very good. However, if you want to do some calculations yourself, you can quite easily figure out how much of a particular nutrient you are adding to an area of land. Remember that fertilizer bags have an analysis written on them that corresponds to the percentage of nitrogen, phosphorus, and potassium that is in the fertilizer. Recommendations on the quantity of fertilizer to apply are usually based on the amount of nitrogen being added since that is the element most responsible for stimulating growth. If you want to apply 2 pounds of nitrogen as a slow-release or granular fertilizer, simply divide 2 pounds by the percent N in your fertilizer and multiply the answer by 100. The result will tell you how many pounds of fertilizer you must apply in order to apply 2 pounds of nitrogen.

For grass, adding 1 to 2 pounds of nitrogen per 1000 square feet is typical. This amount also works well for trees, shrubs, perennials, and annuals. The greater the amount of nitrogen you add, the more likely you are to get rapid growth and the more likely you are to damage your plants. There is rarely a need for anything greater than 2 pounds of nitrogen per 1000 square feet, especially if you have incorporated compost into your soil.

Fertilizer is applied at various times of the year depending on what you are growing. Fertilizer companies often recommend fertilizing grass three times a year, but if you only do it once, early fall is the best time. Grass collects nutrition during early fall to give itself a boost in the spring. By fertilizing it at that time, you are getting it ready to handle the winter. Fertilizing in late fall is not a good idea because you could stimulate tender new growth, which could not handle the winter.

For trees and shrubs the best time to fertilize is usually in early spring. This is when they do most of their growing and will need the most nutrition. Some people recommend fall fertilization, which has some distinct advantages but also some drawbacks. The advantage is that nutrients that are not very mobile in the soil, such as phosphorus and potassium, will be incorporated much better in the fall than in the spring because winter rain and snow will have a chance to move them into the soil. The disadvantage is that nitrogen may move through the soil before the tree or shrub has a chance to take it up. Additionally, if the application is made early enough in the fall so that the tree is still growing, the nitrogen could actually stimulate new growth on the tree. If you live where winter temperatures dip below freezing, this could well result in a loss of new growth as the winter comes. Fertilizer is usually best applied right before a rain or a watering and when it is not too hot outside. Water and cooler temperatures help to reduce the chance of burning the plants.

Which fertilizer to use?

We have worked out the basics of when to fertilize and how to fertilize; it is time to figure out what fertilizer to use. There are all kinds of options, but for my money I'll buy organic fertilizers. Yes, they are more expensive, and yes, because of their low analyses, organic fertilizers need to be applied in heavier doses than synthetic fertilizers. They also, however, release nutrients more slowly than synthetics, are less likely to burn your plants, are a renewable resource, and usually offer micronutrients. If you're keeping score that's 4 to 2—organic fertilizers win. I like to use a fertilizer high in nitrogen, low in phosphorus, and midrange in potassium. Something with a ratio of 5-1-2 should be about right for most situations. If you're growing fruits or vegetables, you may want a little more potassium, and if you're trying to encourage a plant to put on a lot of growth, I'd go with a higher level of nitrogen. The only time that I would use a high level of phosphorus is if I knew for sure that my garden soil was devoid of it or if I was planting grass seed. Even then I would rarely add something with a ratio of nitrogen-phosphorus-potassium any greater than 2-1-1.

If you end up deciding that synthetic fertilizers with higher concentrations of nutrients are right for your situation, good for you. There is absolutely nothing wrong with these fertilizers. I personally like to use a synthetic slow-release fertilizer when growing shrubs and trees in containers because of its cost and convenience. Remember, though, that many synthetic fertilizers do not include all the micronutrients that organic fertilizers do, so if the one you are using does not, consider supplementing it, especially if you are growing plants in containers. Adding micronutrient mixes is certainly an option here, but eggshells (or other foods) boiled in water could also be used to provide some of the micronutrients lacking in the fertilizer. Irrigating plants with water that has some nutrition in it can be a good idea as long as the water doesn't contain so much salt that it hurts the plant. This is rarely an issue unless you really like to salt your water when you boil eggs or vegetables.

3

Water

W ATER IS a valuable resource and one that is too often taken for granted. Every living creature on this planet needs water to live, and plants are certainly no exception. But how much water does a plant need? Should its roots be drenched or do we need to moderate the water that gets to our plant's roots? Is there any way to reduce the need for watering to save time and energy? Gardeners have asked themselves these questions for years, and industries have been more than happy to come up with tools and techniques that supposedly benefit your plants' water relations. But which tools and techniques are really effective and which aren't?

Antitranspirants

These products are usually made of wax, or something similar, and are sprayed onto leaves to prevent a plant from losing water through its foliage. Clogging plant pores is supposed to be good for transplanting and preventing winter injury or if you just want to avoid watering for a few weeks! I would pay a fortune (if I had one) to find out how the inventor of antitranspirants came up with this idea. I would try to contact him or her personally, but that probably isn't possible since antitranspirants have been used since the 1920s (Neilson 1928). Perhaps it all started when someone noticed that they perspired less after using an antiperspirant. If they perspired less, then they needed to drink less to stay hydrated—Hey! That ought to work for a plant too! All we need to do is clog up its pores and we're ready to roll! But does it really get the job done?

The practice

Antitranspirants are typically waxy compounds that are mixed with water and applied to the leaves of trees, shrubs, perennials, or other crops. Application is usually done with a sprayer. Good coverage is very important for antitranspirants, as we count on the pores' being completely covered for the desired results to occur. Some chemicals actually force the plant to close its pores instead of just clogging them, but the use of these compounds is not widespread.

The theory

Antitranspirants really are just like antiperspirants. They are intended to clog the pores, called stomata, of the treated plant to stop water from leaving. And if water loss is stopped, so the theory goes, plants will have less stress during times of transplanting and drought. Antitranspirants have also been suggested to increase a plant's ability to resist winter injury and diseases.

The real story

Antitranspirants have long been a fascination of mine because I have a difficult time figuring out why someone would think it's a good idea to block a normal plant process. Then again, I have the same question about antiperspirants. Yes, I use them, but I'm not completely sold on their safety—it just doesn't seem right to block a natural function like perspiration for any length of time. This leads to very important questions: How long and how effectively can antitranspirants block pores? And how would other pore-blocking products, such as antiperspirants, stack up? With these questions running around in my mind, I decided to investigate the effects of antitranspirants and antiperspirants on plant pores.

In my lab we tested two antiperspirants: unscented Right Guard spray-on and unscented Secret roll-on. We applied these to dogwoods in exactly the same way you would apply them under your arm, and we compared them to two different concentrations (2.5 percent and 10 percent) of a commercial antitranspirant, as well as to a set of plants that were not treated (our control). Using a porometer, we measured how effective these products were at blocking transpiration. A porometer forms a seal around a small area on a leaf and continuously samples the humidity within that small space in order to measure how open the pores of a plant are. If the pores are wide open, water will easily move from the interior of the leaf into the atmosphere, and the humidity should be high. If the pores are mostly shut or blocked, water will have trouble exiting the leaf and the humidity should be low.

We took porometer readings every 2 days for a week. Originally we had intended to continue testing these products for longer, but by the end of the week the results painted a clear picture. None of the products sampled lasted longer than a week in terms of their ability to slow water movement out of the plants' leaves. In the short term (2 days) the best product was, by far, Secret. Secret blocked nearly two-thirds of the water loss that the control plant experienced. The Right Guard and both concentrations of antitranspirant prevented nearly half the water loss. Four days after the treatment, we detected no difference. It is worth noting that plants treated with Secret did show some leaf distortion, including some curling and wrinkling, indicating that this product was somewhat toxic to the plant.

The results of our small experiment indicate that antitranspirants are pretty useless products for plants; fortunately, we are not the only source of data out there (unless you count using the Secret and Right Guard in which case we probably are). Indeed, some research has shown that these products do have their uses. Most of the published research on antitranspirants investigates their ability to aid plant survival and health during a brief time of high stress, such as transplanting. Under transplant conditions large plants such as photinias, azaleas, and small trees showed some benefit when antitranspirants were used (Ponder at al. 1983; Ceulemans et al. 1983; Englert et al. 1993). However, when smaller plants, such as impatiens, were tested, results clearly showed that antitranspirants offered no benefit (van Iersel 1998a).

Although stopping a tree from transpiring may certainly have benefits in and of itself, antitranspirants have been reported to offer other, less likely benefits, including increased cold tolerance and disease protection. Research investigating the ability of antitranspirants to protect peppers and tomatoes from cold showed this practice provided little benefit (Perry et al. 1992). They also didn't do much to protect peaches from freezing (Aoun et al. 1993), but they did increase the storage life of sycamore kept in cold rooms (Filer and Nelson 1987).

Water loss over the winter months can claim a plant's life just as readily as absolute cold can. Plants usually suffer more from desiccation over the winter than from cold temperatures because, when the ground is frozen, trees cannot pull water from the soil. With the inability to pull water from the soil and the cold, dry winds of winter whipping through their branches (and leaves in the case of evergreens), plants tend to lose a lot of water without replenishing it. It stands to reason that covering a plant with a waxy coating would prevent some water loss. Unfortunately, based on our small trial and on other research, antitranspirants don't last long enough to really have an effect on winter desiccation—unless you live in Hawaii.

Most research shows that winter protection just isn't the best use of antitranspirants, but disease protection is a different story entirely. Even partially covering a leaf's surface with a coating might help to protect that leaf from the clutches of all kinds of nasty diseases; indeed, that is just what the research shows. The severity of downy mildew in cucumbers (Haggag 2002) and powdery mildew in dogwoods (Mmbaga and Sheng 2002) may be reduced by the application of antitranspirants, and it is likely that other diseases could be controlled and other plants could benefit from applications of these products as well.

What it means to you ❀❀❀

Antitranspirants may be useful in certain circumstances, but they certainly aren't a miracle cure. These are the wrong products for reducing the need to water. Antitranspirants simply will not block the pores of a plant for a long-enough time to be effective. This inability also makes these products ineffective at reducing water loss over winter months.

For transplanting, mixed results are present, but in a situation where a high-value tree is to be moved, an antitranspirant is probably worth a try: it could help and is unlikely to do much harm. Applications of these products are unlikely to improve cold hardiness or relieve damage caused by winter but may provide some control of diseases. Now, I wonder how antiperspirants would work for disease control.

Gravel for drainage ❦

We all know that plants like good drainage. If water is allowed to sit around the roots of a plant for too long, root rot will ensue, which will at best damage the plant and at worst kill the plant. For plants in containers, an accepted practice has been to cover the bottom of the container with gravel, oyster shells, or some other nonabsorbent material so that more water will drain out of the container and keep the plant roots moist instead of wet. Despite my best efforts I cannot figure out where or when this practice began, but I can tell you that it was a recommended technique in the early 1900s. An article in *House and Garden* suggested it as a beneficial way to make a container more inviting for plants (Edson 1917).

The practice

Oyster shells, large diameter gravel, rocks, pieces of pottery, and other nonabsorbent things are placed in the bottom of the container, from one-eighth up to one-half of the depth. After these are added, the rest of the container is filled up with more-typical potting media.

The theory

Because the nonabsorbent material at the bottom of the container will not hold much water, it makes sense to some people that the media will drain better if this material is added.

The real story

Dr. Mark Rieger at the University of Georgia elegantly dispelled for me the myth of using gravel in the base of a container to improve drainage. Lay a rectangular sponge flat on your hand and saturate it with water. Wait until the excess water has dripped out (maybe 15 seconds). The sponge is fully saturated. Now turn the sponge 90 degrees so it is upright, with the long side of the sponge perpendicular to the floor. What happened? Water leaked out, right? That is because the shape of a container actually has a lot to do with how much water the container holds. A round, shallow container filled with media will hold more water per unit area than a container that has a similar diameter but is longer. Since drainage has everything to do with how much water a container will hold per unit area, the longer container will drain better.

When you are adding media to the top of the gravel you are effectively making a container that is shallower than it was intended to be. Although this container will hold less total water than a similar container filled entirely with media, the top section of the container, where there should be much root growth (the section without the gravel), will actually hold more water per unit area than the same section in a container filled entirely with media. Additionally, the water in the upper portion of the container does not move easily from a layer of finer-textured material to a layer of more course-textured material, compounding the drainage problem. Conclusion? Water drainage is actually better if you just fill your container all the way with potting media.

What it means to you ❀

Don't use gravel or other nonabsorbent materials at the bottom of your container to increase drainage. If you feel you need better drainage simply buy better-draining media from your local garden center. If you still feel you need better drainage you might consider adding some perlite, a commercial media amendment available at most garden centers.

Hydrogels

Some people love to go out and water their plants, and for some people watering is a drag. I must admit that, for me, the fun is in the plants themselves and not in the watering. Houseplants are especially tiresome as they require you not only to water the plant but also to avoid watering nearby things that may not like to get wet, such as the carpet, wall, or family dog. Fortunately, modern science has created a series of products that will absorb water and supposedly release it to a plant over time, thereby reducing the need for watering and potentially even increasing plant health. These products are called hydrogels. Hydrogels are whitish or clear crystals about the size of large sugar grains before they are introduced to water. Once they absorb water they look like amorphous masses of clear Jell-O. The first modern hydrogels were introduced when Richard Herrett and Paul King, who worked for Union Carbide at the time, received a patent in 1967 (which they applied for in 1963) called simply "Plant Growth Medium." The patent was for a group of chemical compounds that were supposed to "reversibly sorb and desorb substantial amounts of liquids."

The practice

Commercial hydrogels are suggested for use either in containers or on bare soil. Application rates and instructions are listed on the label and usually consist of a few teaspoons or tablespoons of hydrogel crystals per pot, depending on pot size. It is generally recommended to incorporate these products into the growing media or soil before planting to ensure water is evenly available to the plant's roots throughout the mixture.

The theory

The idea behind hydrogels is that they will absorb water during times of excess, store the water until it is needed by the plant, and then release it during times of drought.

The real story

Hydrogels can hold over 600 times their weight in water, but this water is not necessarily transferred to the plant, as the companies selling these products would have you believe. In our lab we looked at a few different hydrogels and their abilities to reduce the need for watering. We tested five different hydrogels on geranium (grown in large flower pots) and three different hydrogels on ninebark (grown in gallon containers) to see how long we could keep the plants healthy without watering.

The plants were grown in containers and treated with hydrogels from a very young age until they filled the containers and would have been large and lush enough for a typical homeowner to buy. They were irrigated whenever the media in the container was less than 80 percent saturated with water. (We weighed all the containers to figure this out—when the container was 80 percent of its maximum post-watering weight, more water was added.) After most of the plants reached a size that was considered saleable, watering was stopped and the plants were allowed to dry out. The amount of water in the plants themselves was determined by using a "pressure bomb," an instrument that measures how much water is in a leaf by compressing the leaf with air until sap comes out of the petiole (base of the leaf). The more pressure that needs to be applied, the less water in the plant tissue. Plant growth was roughly similar among the control and the different hydrogels tested, with the exception of one, Hydrosorb. It stunted the growth of the ninebark. The results showed that none of the hydrogels kept the plants supplied with water any longer than plants grown with nothing added to the media. It is worth mentioning that the hydrogel that stunted the plants' growth did appear to keep them at a healthy water potential for longer than the other hydrogels and the control. However, because of the smaller size of the plants, they would lose less water through transpiration and therefore use less water (Gillman 2004).

Research by other scientists has shown results that are pretty similar. In a test on tropical ornamental plants, hydrogels either didn't extend the time to wilting or only extended the time by about 12 percent—from 24 to 27 days (Wang 1989). Other experiments using privets and azaleas demonstrated that hydrogels are not particularly effective in reducing the number of times that watering has to be conducted (Keever et al. 1989). The same results were found in experiments on birch trees grown in containers with hydrogels added (Tripepi et al. 1991). In a more recent study conducted on highly drought-sensitive plants, such as petunia, grown in landscape beds, hydrogels did prove to be somewhat beneficial (Boatright et al. 1997). But generally, reports indicate that hydrogels aren't particularly helpful in reducing watering frequency.

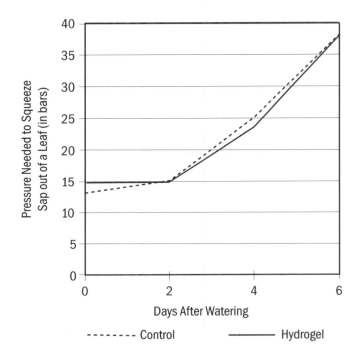

Figure 5. The effectiveness of one hydrogel at keeping ninebark hydrated as compared to no amendment. Plants showed signs of wilting at around 25 bars. Various hydrogels were tested, but none fared better than the one illustrated here.

What it means to you ❋❋

In most cases hydrogels just don't work very well. While these products have shown themselves somewhat useful in some tests, they haven't proven themselves on a consistent basis, and when they have reduced watering frequency, they haven't reduced it by much.

There is one application where these gels can be counted on to be effective. When removing a plant from the ground without including any soil on the roots for transplant, some people like to fill a bucket with hydrogels and water and dip the roots of the removed plant into this bucket. The hydrogels will stick to the roots and help prevent them from drying out when they are removed from the bucket and moved to the location where they are to be planted (as long as the move is a short distance).

Planting deeply 🌱

"Everyone knows that if you leave the roots on the surface of the soil they'll just dry out. You've got to plant deep to keep them moist." So said an old neighbor of mine who subsequently lost most of the trees he planted. Back in 1618 William Lawson stated that trees should never be planted deeply for fear of injury, and ever since, gardeners, academics, and foresters have argued this idea back and forth.

The practice

Those who recommend planting deeply suggest digging a hole that is deep enough for a few inches of soil to cover the uppermost root on the plant. The tree or shrub is then placed in this hole and the hole is filled with soil so it covers not only the root system, but also the bottom few inches of the stem.

The theory

People who plant their trees deeply adhere to the theory that since there is more water in the ground the deeper you dig then it must be good to plant deeply to get as much water as possible around the roots. People who plant deeply also tend to believe that increasing the depth of their planting will help to prevent newly planted trees from being knocked over by the wind.

The real story

Planting deeply to get the roots of your plants into better contact with water can backfire on you, and it frequently does. Plant roots grow toward a balance of air and water; if they have too much water they will die. Alternatively, if the plants don't die, their roots will grow upward to get the air they are lacking. While growing upward, these roots seem to lose their orientation and sometimes grow across the plant's stem. This causes a problem. When a plant's roots and a plant's stem compete, the stem loses. Over time, as the roots and stem grow, the stem will become constricted by the crossing roots, and the tree will literally strangle itself to death.

Studies investigating the effects of planting apple trees deeply show that these trees tend to be less stable than trees planted at a shallower depth, as well as having smaller leaves and thinner trunks (Lyons et al. 1982; Lyons et al. 1983). Other more recent studies by Gary Johnson and Ben Johnson (2000), two leaders in planting-depth research, show that urban street trees that have roots wrapping around their stems are more likely to have been planted deeply, making them less stable and more likely to fall over in a storm.

Herbaceous plants like tomatoes and peppers seem to be able to handle somewhat-deeper planting than trees. These plants can easily produce new roots from their lower stems, so while planting deeply might not be the best thing for them, it's not the worst either.

What it means to you ❀

Deep planting might get your tree more water, but this is likely to backfire in the long run because of drowned roots or roots that girdle the stem and strangle the tree to death. You may need to water your tree a little more for the first month or two if you plant shallowly, but you will be saving yourself a lot of trouble in the future. Plants in general and trees in particular need to be planted properly. When a tree is planted, its roots should be just barely visible at ground level around the trunk. Mulch should be added but should not touch the stem because roots can grow up into the mulch and surround the stem just as they can in soil.

Sponges for water retention

Some garden gurus seem to think they can find things in their homes that will substitute for hydrogels. Considering what we now know about hydrogels, I would say it is a good bet they can. Having seen recommendations for using sponges as a hydrogel substitute, I thought it would be worthwhile to see whether they could lengthen the time between waterings for a plant.

The practice

Simply chop up a sponge and mix it with your media before planting. Little data is available indicating the amount of sponge to use, but we used 50 cubic inches of chopped up synthetic sponge per gallon of media.

The theory

As with hydrogels, the sponges are supposed to collect water during times of excess and release it during times of need.

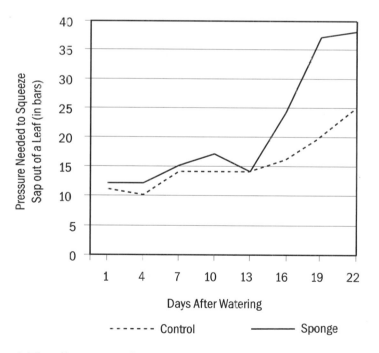

Figure 6. The effectiveness of sponges at retaining water for butterfly bushes growing in containers. Media without sponges is better for keeping plants hydrated.

The real story

Because of the lack of research on this subject I took it upon myself to take this home remedy for a test drive. We tested butterfly bushes grown in 1-gallon containers with no amendment (our control) against plants that were grown in similar containers with a chopped up sponge added. After growing the plants for a few weeks, we ceased watering and measured the water potential of the leaves every 3 days as the plants dried out. The procedure was similar to the test of hydrogels.

Because the plants were relatively small and were growing in relatively large containers, they took a long time to dry out. At the end of the first week after we had stopped watering, some real differences were apparent. By the third week, most plants with sponge in their media were essentially dead, and those with regular media, while not healthy, were certainly not dead. The results painted a clear picture about using sponges for water retention. It isn't effective.

What it means to you ❀

After testing the sponges, I'm tempted to say they might actually be good for improving the drainage of media. They surely don't increase the amount of water available to plants.

Putting it all together

As we have seen, all kinds of home-brewed remedies are intended to help you get water to your plants' roots. Some obviously work better than others, but the best practice is to plant correctly so that roots are in the right location to intercept the proper amount of water and air.

It all starts with proper planting

Planting properly is very important. The root crown should be even with the surface of the soil or media. This will ensure that roots grow in the direction they're supposed to—down rather than up, which may cause problems.

The type of plant can have a significant effect on the amount of water you need to apply. Since plants take up water through their roots, plants with larger root systems need less frequent watering because they will be able to scrounge water for themselves, and those with smaller root systems will need to be irrigated quite frequently. Plants that are purchased in containers are usually planted into your garden with most of their roots intact. While they certainly need to be watered frequently at first, they will soon spread their roots out and be able to fend for themselves. Plants not purchased in containers generally need a longer period of time before they can efficiently capture their own water. Trees are often purchased as balled-and-burlapped stock. This type of harvest usually means that anywhere from 70 to 90 percent of the plant's root mass has been removed; these plants need quite a bit of attention their first year to ensure that they receive enough water. Houseplants are not even as fortunate as balled-and-burlapped plants because they constantly need watering. The plants are limited by the volume of water their container holds rather than by the size of their root system. If they use up everything in their container, they're out of luck until more is added.

When and how to water

The best technique I have found for watering is to turn the hose on to a slow trickle and saturate the ground or container where your plants are growing. This saturation is more than your plants need, but if your soil or media has good drainage, air will soon move into it to create optimal growth conditions. These conditions will last for a variable amount of time, depending on the drainage of your media and the weather conditions your plant is exposed to. Although different circumstances call for different watering regimes, I usually use what is commonly known as the "finger test" to determine when my plants need watering. I put my finger into the soil or media up to the first knuckle; if the soil feels dry and nothing sticks to my finger when I pull it out, then I need to water. If the soil feels moist and soil sticks to my finger when I pull it out, the plants are fine. You could also purchase a soil moisture indicator from your local garden center; they tend to be cheap and to work well.

Adding appropriate amendments

Amendments that provide extra water when plants need it would be a boon, especially with balled-and-burlapped plants that are about to be transplanted or with plants growing in containers. Unfortunately, amendments that reduce the need for frequent watering have proved to be a waste of time in most situations. Hydrogels may increase the amount of time that water is available, but this benefit cannot be relied upon, based on the divergent results of various studies. You can be sure that chopping sponges and placing them in your media will do absolutely nothing for increasing the amount of water available to your plants.

Amendments for drainage are not a bad idea, but adding gravel to the bottom of your container will actually make drainage worse as well as decrease the amount of water your container will hold. In outdoor situations, compost usually helps drainage. It improves both the water retention and aeration of soils, so when you add it to help fertility, you will also improve your soil's water relations. If you are growing in containers and feel that increasing drainage is a priority, buy a premade container mix with good drainage, or buy perlite and add it to the mix you are already using. Vermiculite will not be as effective as perlite because vermiculite tends to break down over time.

Beyond the soil and media, little can be done to affect a plant's water relations. Coatings applied to plant leaves for conserving water wear off rapidly. They can, however, be effective at improving plant survival when applied at the time of transplanting. Coatings may also offer the plant some protection from disease.

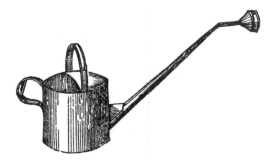

4

Biostimulants

ONCOCTIONS to increase the health, growth, and yield of your vegetables, trees, shrubs, and roses are on the shelves of every garden center. The concoctions aren't just fertilizers, either; they're also biostimulants. What is a biostimulant? It is loosely defined as a non-fertilizer that, when applied to a plant, will result in a modification of plant growth. Indeed, plants can only grow as much as the water and nutrition in their environment will allow, but biostimulants are supposed to maximize a plant's ability to utilize resources or to redirect resources to produce growth in a particular area, such as the roots. Many biostimulants are available on the market today, and some you can make yourself. Most of the ones you buy contain one, two, or three of the products listed in this chapter, mixed in a concoction that can be either applied directly to the plant or mixed with water and applied to the soil around the plant. Most biostimulants also contain some fertilizer; the question is whether biostimulants will produce growth that is more than or different from what could be obtained with fertilizers alone. It would be easy to say that all biostimulants are just smoke and mirrors, but the truth is that some have been shown to have real value in certain situations.

Humic acids

Humic acids are one of the biostimulants most touted to have a positive effect on your plants. They come from a variety of sources, but are most commonly extracted from leonardite, which is a brownish-black form of coal. They have been reported to increase the growth and health of various plants, especially plants in stressful situations.

The practice

An incredible variety of humic acid products are for sale, with numerous recommended concentrations and methods of application, depending on the product purchased. Hence, there is no standard application method; the instructions offered on the product you purchase need to be followed.

The theory

It's tough to figure out what the companies selling this stuff think humic acids do to make plants healthier—little agreement exists between the companies trying to hawk these products. The most common claim is that humic acids will have auxin-like effects on plants, but we also see claims that they help RNA production, increase chlorophyll content, hinder disease, increase nutrient uptake, and do a host of other things. Most of these claims don't make much sense and are hard to understand anyway, so let's put them aside for now and take a look at some more-trustworthy scientific sources that paint a different picture.

The real story

Research on humic acids is somewhat more complete than the research for the other biostimulants, except for mycorrhizae, IBA, and NAA. Humic acids have been shown to be beneficial to plant growth in some cases, not beneficial in others, and possibly even detrimental to plant growth in certain situations (De Kreij and Basar 1995). This confusing list of possible results certainly explains why humic acids are not products we see every day.

Let's first take a closer look at the claim that applying humic acids will have auxin-like effects. This claim is important because auxins are a naturally occurring group of hormones found in all plants. These hormones do promote growth, especially root growth, and can enhance the ability of a plant to survive when it is faced with adverse conditions such as transplanting (Scagel and Linderman 2001). In fact, auxins are typically used to promote roots in plant cuttings during propagation (Dirr and Heuser 1987). (See the entry "Indole-3-butyric acid and naphthalene-3-acetic acid".) If indeed present, auxin-like properties certainly could have an effect on plants and should not be discounted.

While interesting, the evidence for auxin-like effects is somewhat shaky. Tests on pea plants show that humic acid promotes rooting, but the researchers who conducted this study noted that "the root of the pea plant is extremely sensitive to auxins," (O'Donnell 1973) meaning that the level of auxin-like activity could have been ineffective on anything but a pea plant. This is kind of like saying that because an electric motor can run a child's toy car it can also run a tractor trailer. This may be true, but it is unlikely. More evidence needs to be presented before I'll believe it.

Humic acids are more likely to benefit a plant through their ability to increase nutrient availability in the soil by forming chelates with elements in the soil and hence allowing those elements to be absorbed by plants at a wide variety of pH levels. These chelates benefit plants growing in conditions where they have trouble collecting various nutrients because the soil pH is too high. In experiments testing nutrient uptake, humic acids proved beneficial to the uptake of iron and other elements (Adani et al. 1998), but whether humic acids would be more beneficial than commercially available chelates is in doubt.

What it means to you ❀❀❀

Biostimulants based on humic acid really aren't a bad idea if you know that your soil conditions are alkaline and that your plants prefer more acidic conditions. Plants in this situation can use all the iron they can get, and the chelating abilities of humic acid may very well help out (of course you could just buy some iron chelate). Do not expect miracles, but a moderate benefit is a possibility. If your plants are sited properly, however, there is little reason to believe that humic acids will help your cause. Biostimulants in general and humic acids in particular seem to be most useful for plants under stress, and most research showing these chemicals to be beneficial has been conducted on plants under stress. Non-stressed plants tend not to respond to these products, so if you're growing a healthy garden, watering when needed, planting the right plants for your soil type, and fertilizing, humic acids are probably a waste of time.

Indole-3-butyric acid and naphthalene-3-acetic acid 🌱

Most root-stimulating products on the garden center shelves contain mysterious chemicals named indole-3-butyric acid (IBA) and naphthalene-3-acetic acid (NAA). These chemicals are packaged and marketed to do one of two things: to promote rooting of cuttings or to stimulate root formation in newly planted trees, shrubs, and other plants.

Many experienced gardeners like to propagate their own plants rather than buy them. They have many different options available, but if they want to produce a plant that does not differ from its parent, they will use vegetative propagation. Vegetative propagation involves cutting and treating a portion of the parent plant (other than the seed) in a way that promotes root and shoot formation. This practice is most commonly carried out with sections of stem.

Certain plants, including grapes, blackberries, figs, and olives, have been propagated vegetatively for thousands of years, but the real breakthrough occurred in 1935 when Thimann and Koepfli discovered that when an auxin was applied to a cutting (usually a stem cutting), root growth would often ensue. IBA and NAA are chemicals closely related to those that Thimann and Koepfli used in their original experiments.

The practice

To root cuttings using IBA or NAA, a gardener should purchase a propagation guide—the intricacies of using these hormones are well beyond the scope of this book. Two recommended guides are Michael Dirr's and Charles Heuser's *The Reference Manual of Woody Plant Propagation* (1987) and Bruce MacDonald's *Practical Woody Plant Propagation for Nursery Growers* (1986).

Commercial products utilize IBA or NAA to encourage root growth. The concentration of these chemicals in different products varies, so the instructions on the label need to be closely followed.

The theory

IBA and NAA are auxins. Auxins in general, and these auxins in particular, have been used to encourage root production for many years. They are supposed to accomplish this by making the plant cells react as if they were root cells. The idea that these compounds can be used to promote further root production in plants that already have roots, however, is a relatively new one.

The real story

From personal tests and experience I can, without reservation, say that IBA and NAA are effective chemicals for stimulating root production from stem cuttings and that, without these chemicals, producing roots where none would normally grow is extremely difficult if not impossible in some species. But what about claims that they will stimulate root production on recently harvested plants with a small root system? If a plant already has roots can IBA or NAA stimulate more? And if more roots are produced does that mean the plant will be more likely to survive when it is planted out?

Adding IBA and NAA to plants' roots before they are planted has been shown to increase root growth in hackberry (Tuskan and Ellis 1991) and to benefit both root growth and transplant survival in a number of trees, including black walnut, Douglas fir, scarlet oak, and tulip poplar (Scagel et al. 2000; Struve et al. 1983). For some trees, including little leaf linden and Colorado blue spruce, use of IBA is more effective in the fall than in the spring (Lumis 1987; Carter and Tripepi 1989).

Despite these success stories, IBA and NAA do not always promote roots, and experiments have been conducted that showed no increased root growth for a number of trees, such as common birch, ponderosa pine, red oak, and sugar maple (Lumis 1987; Struve and Joly 1992; Tuskan and Ellis 1991). Bedding plants, such as petunia and impatiens, also seem to be less responsive to IBA and other root enhancers (van Iersel 1998a).

What it means to you

For producing roots on cuttings ✿✿✿✿✿. IBA and NAA have a very positive effect on rooting cuttings; in many cases rooting would be impossible without them. They won't provide miracles, however, and every attempt will not be successful just because these chemicals are used. But the use of IBA and NAA, along with a good propagation guide, will greatly increase your ability to vegetatively propagate plants.

For stimulating root growth on material to be transplanted ✿✿✿. Using products containing IBA or NAA for transplanting can be a good idea, but it doesn't always work, is less likely to work in the spring than in the fall, and is less likely to work on smaller herbaceous plants than on trees and shrubs. It was a toss-up between three and four flowerheads for this product, but I went with three because the companies that produce these mixtures make claims that are just a little too extravagant. Nonetheless, these chemicals do seem beneficial, especially for someone planting trees in the fall.

Mycorrhizal myths

Mycorrhizae have become all the rage. They are fungi that live symbiotically with plants (in other words, both organisms, the plant and the fungi, benefit from living together) and are marketed as being beneficial to a plant's nutrient uptake and disease resistance. These fabulous fungi live in almost all soils, so is it worth adding extra to your garden?

The practice

Mycorrhizae are usually mixed with a carrier, such as peat, that keeps them moist and dilutes them so they can easily be applied at the correct concentration. This mixture is then worked into the soil, at which point the mycorrhizae are supposed to grow onto your plants' root surface.

The theory

Essentially, mycorrhizae are supposed to provide extra "roots" for a plant by attaching to the plant's existing roots and spreading out across the soil. While spreading, the mycorrhizae are supposed to pick up nutrients that the plant might miss out on, primarily phosphorus. In return, the plant offers the mycorrhizae some of the carbohydrates that it produces through photosynthesis.

The real story

There is no doubt that naturally occurring mycorrhizae are beneficial to many plants (Raven et al. 1986). The question is whether additions of store-bought mycorrhizae are beneficial.

In situations where a lot of fertilizer is likely to be added to the plant, mycorrhizae are unlikely to help. Mycorrhizae normally scrounge for nutrients in the soil, and plants use these nutrients (among other things) to create sugars that it shares with the mycorrhizae. Under conditions of high nutrition the plant does not need help from the mycorrhizae to find nutrients; the mycorrhizae become superfluous and could, in some cases, even inhibit a plant's growth because the plant is giving up sugars without getting anything substantial in return. In this case the mycorrhizae could actually be considered parasites (Buwalda and Goh 1982; Johnson et al. 1992). Mycorrhizae are best at scrounging phosphorus. In general, if much phosphorus is provided by fertilizers, mycorrhizae will not be able to colonize plants as effectively (Linderman and Davis 2004; Olsen et al. 1996).

Overkill is another issue to consider. Many studies demonstrate that mycorrhizae are beneficial, but these studies tend to look at sterilized soil, where there is little chance that any mycorrhizal spores are present. If mycorrhizal spores are present, as in the case with most garden soils, it is likely that they will colonize any plant in the area—addition of new spores is unnecessary. It is also possible that commercial mycorrhizae are not the best mycorrhizae for the job. Many different types of mycorrhizae exist, and commercial formulations are certainly not the only appropriate mycorrhizae for your garden, if they contain appropriate mycorrhizae at all. Indeed, the mycorrhizae that are best for your conditions are probably already in your soil.

Finally, and perhaps most importantly, living mycorrhizae may or may not be present in a mycorrhizal mix that you buy at the garden center. Mycorrhizae are fairly susceptible to extremes in environmental conditions, such as temperature. If the garden center or shipper did a bad job of storing the containers, you may be purchasing nothing but a little bit of peat and some dead spores.

What it means to you ❀❀❀

If you purchase mycorrhizae that are alive, if you are not fertilizing much, and if your soil is low in natural mycorrhizae (unlikely in most situations), these fungi may be beneficial to you. Because there are so many types of mycorrhizae and the companies producing them must ensure many plants will benefit, the mycorrhizae you purchase may not even be the type that is best for the plants you care about. In short, adding mycorrhizae may be beneficial in a few circumstances, but as a general practice adding these fungi to your soil or media is not particularly useful.

Seaweed extracts

Seaweed extract is just that—seaweed with most of the solid portions removed. As far as I can tell, seaweed extracts are supposed to provide benefits to plants simply because they are seaweed. I think a deeper look is in order.

The practice

Like humic acids, seaweed extract is available in a wide variety of concoctions and so it is impossible to describe all the ways that it might be applied to a plant to encourage additional growth, but seaweed extracts are most commonly applied as a foliar spray or as a soil application. When these products are used the directions should be followed closely to avoid damaging plants.

The theory

This extract is commonly reported to contain vitamins and minerals that improve plant health, as well as cytokinins and auxins, two plant hormones that might benefit plant growth in certain circumstances.

The real story

Research on seaweed extracts is in its infancy at best. Some studies have shown that seaweed extracts provide benefits to some plants, especially when the plants are under stress (Zhang et al. 2003a,). Other studies have shown that seaweed extracts do not help plants, even when stress is present (Elliot and Prevatte 1996). The studies swing back and forth, and it's tough to get a firm grasp on whether products containing seaweed will be helpful; sometimes they seem to work and sometimes they don't. So, let's take a step back and look at some of the research.

Seaweed extracts have been reported to contain plant hormones, including cytokinins and auxins (Sanderson and Jameson 1986; Crouch et al. 1992). Cytokinins encourage plant cell elongation. Auxins encourage growth, particularly root growth. It is no surprise, in and of itself, that seaweed contains these hormones. We expect seaweed, being a plant, to contain all the hormones that surface-dwelling plants do. The important question is whether seaweed has extraordinary amounts of these hormones. If seaweed extracts do contain high levels of auxins and cytokinins, there certainly is a chance that they might benefit root growth. When researchers tried to quantify the amount of cytokinin in seaweed extract, they found that, though this hormone is present, it may be at one-hundredth the concentration claimed by the company selling the extract (Sanderson and Jameson 1986). When the amount of auxin was examined, the concentration was in one case roughly similar to what would be found in regular, surface-dwelling plants (Sanderson et al. 1987). In a separate case concentrations of auxin were quite high (Kingman and Moore 1982). So which tests are correct? What to believe? I wish I knew. Perhaps the difference in hormone levels mirrors the difference in responses that researchers see when they try these extracts on various crops.

Seaweed extracts will certainly offer some nutrients simply because they come from living plants. These nutrients will help the plant the same as any fertilizer, but anything beyond that is uncertain based on the research that is out there.

What it means to you ✿✿

Seaweed extracts do not seem to be a particularly valuable addition to the gardener's palette. Although they may provide some benefit under certain circumstances, the variable results that scientists have had when trying seaweed extracts make it impossible to predict exactly when this stuff will work and when it won't. It's also hard to tell whether benefits realized from extracts are due to hormones or simply to the nutrition that the extracts provide. As with humic acids, these products are supposed to be more effective when plants are stressed. Application of seaweed extracts won't usually hurt anything if they are used as indicated on the instructions, so if you want to spend your money on something that may or may not benefit your plants, this is certainly as good a purchase as any. For me, I'll stick with spending my money on fertilizers and hoses, two things I know will work and will hopefully keep me from having stressed plants in the first place.

Sound for plants ❦

Not all biostimulants are solids or liquids; some are less tangible. Promoting good health in plants through speaking, playing an instrument, or using a sound generator is not a new idea, but it is one that has found a great deal of support. Way back in 1848 a German by the name of Gustav Theodor Fechner pronounced that, though plants do not have a nervous system like we do, they may still have emotions (1909). Even today some people think that talking to, or playing music for, their plants will make them healthier. These people are nuts, right?

The practice

Sound is used to stimulate growth in two ways. The first is to play music (or a single tone) to plants, and the second is to play sounds to plants while at the same time applying fertilizers to the foliage. The music or sounds can be applied at a variety of frequencies and volumes, but higher frequencies have been reported by some to work better, and rock music has been reported to be less effective at stimulating growth than classical.

The theory

Most proponents of using sound to encourage plant growth do not claim to know why it works, just that it does. Others, usually those who recommend adding foliar fertilizers at the same time as applying sound, claim that sound will stimulate stomata (pores) on the plant's leaves to open. When fertilizer is applied to leaves that have their stomata wide open, it is supposed to enter the plant with greater ease.

The real story

Scientists of Fechner's time seem to have generally ignored his theories, but in 1973 a book by Peter Tompkins and Christopher Bird, *The Secret Life of Plants*, took a semi-serious look at his ideas. Unfortunately for Fechner, this is probably not where he would have wanted his thoughts to be published. The book relates some fascinating information about plants, including their ability to sense alien beings, read minds, and open doors (with a little help from humans). If I had read it as a child I wouldn't have eaten vegetables for a week, much as children who learn that hamburgers are made from cows may become vegetarians for a day or two. Needless to say, the world of serious science didn't immediately latch on to the ideas presented.

In the same year that Tompkins and Bird published their book, Dorothy Retallack came out with a book titled *The Sound of Music and Plants*. This is a wonderful book written by someone who was not a researcher. Rather, she was a grandmother who attended college late in life, took a class in biology in which she did an interesting project on the effects of music on plants, and published what she found in a book. Her research was not designed properly to be published in scientific journals, but it was well organized and raised some interesting questions. Additionally, she did an excellent job of describing how she conducted her research, making it reproducible by future researchers.

Retallack describes how she played various types of music for plants over long periods of time and observed how this affected their growth. What she found was fascinating. Some types of music, such as easy listening, seemed to promote plant growth while some music, mostly what she called "acid rock" (including such groups as Vanilla Fudge and Led Zeppelin), seemed to hurt plants. But the most interesting thing Retallack noted (at least to me) was that plants exposed to acid rock had to be watered more often than similar plants not exposed to this music. This might indicate that plants open their pores in response to music, resulting in a more rapid loss of moisture through the plants' stomata. Retallack thought of this and ran an experiment with beakers that were filled with water and exposed to different types of music, thereby taking the plants out of the equation. What she found was quite telling. Water in beakers exposed to the rock music evaporated faster than water in beakers exposed to lighter music, which in turn evaporates faster than water in beakers exposed to no music. This occurs because music causes the water to ripple, and the more the water ripples, the more surface area (the amount of water in contact with the air) the water has, leading to faster evaporation. To make the effects of surface area clear to yourself you could take two glasses of water and dump one onto a waterproof floor. The water that has been dumped onto the floor will have a greater surface area than the water still in the glass. You will notice that the water on the floor will evaporate more quickly (over the course of an hour or two) than the water still in the glass because more water is in contact with the air.

After Retallack's work, the next occurrences of consequence are two patents conferred in 1989 and 1991 to Danis Carlson. These patents are for a plant treatment combining the application of a high-pitched tone at a high volume with a fertilizer (or an herbicide). The author of these patents claimed the sound would open the pores of the plant, allowing nutrition, provided by a foliar application of the fertilizer, to be more efficiently absorbed. In his patents Mr. Carlson included a number of examples where this system had been effective, but because these reports are so inexact, it is hard to give them much credence.

All this research leads to many questions but few answers. Though both Retallack's and Carlson's work imply that stomata are affected by music, there is no real evidence in the form of measurements of stomatal conductance (a measurement, taken with a porometer, of stomata openness). Professional researchers have investigated sound and plants, but their research, like that of Carlson's and Retallack's, has been targeted at investigating the effects of sound rather than the cause of these effects. Wheat seedlings have been shown to be affected positively by low-frequency sounds and variably by higher-frequency sounds, which sometimes seem to increase growth and sometimes seem to stunt it (Weryszko-Chmielewska 1990). Other studies that look at bioelectric potentials across leaf surfaces in response to various sounds seem to show that plants are more sensitive to rhythm than tone, but these studies do not really address whether plants will benefit from the sounds, simply that they respond (Miwa et al. 1992).

When I first heard that sound could possibly cause anything substantial to happen, I was skeptical. I really didn't see how music could accomplish this, but I figured if the people who sold sound equipment with foliar fertilizers were right, it would be easy for me to run a simple little experiment to test the theory that music could open a plant's stomata. After all, I have easy access to a porometer, and I have a large number of plants that would no doubt enjoy a serenade. I selected some music that I thought would serve the purpose: Rush. I chose Rush because, for those of you unfamiliar with the popular music of the 1980s, Rush produced a form of rock commonly known as fantasy rock. Had my experiments failed to show that music caused a stomatal response, I could then make an amusing anecdote about fantasies. It now seems that I won't get the chance.

Over the course of 2 weeks on randomly selected days I played either Rush or nothing to radishes. I also took three readings on the porometer at fixed times: morning, noon, and late afternoon. After the data had been collected the results were rather clear. Playing Rush to plants seemed to stimulate them to close their stomata, and here I say "seemed to" because there were other factors, including other sounds, that were present, which could have stimulated stomata to open or close. It is very difficult to control sound in an environment that was not intended for that purpose. On days when we played Rush, the porometer would often show readings only half as high as when nothing was played. Sound stimulating stomata to close makes sense. Noise is naturally caused by the wind blowing, and it may benefit plants to close their stomata under windy conditions to avoid losing excess water. Additionally, because we know from Retallack's work that sound will cause water to evaporate faster, it makes sense that a plant might close its stomata in response to sound to conserve water. But here I am speculating well beyond the evidence. While it is fun to speculate, the truth is that there has not been enough research conducted to convince me that sound can reliably close, or open, stomata or stimulate, or inhibit, plant growth.

What it means to you ?????

So, what if music can affect plants? What does that mean to you? Probably nothing. Plants are going to be subjected to a number of outside stimuli, including music, that you can't control. There is little reason to believe that this incidental music will do much of anything. The fact that fantasy rock seemed to stimulate stomata to close does not indicate that the closure would necessarily be beneficial. Likewise, if stomata are forced open by music there is little to indicate that this necessarily aids the plant in any way. Though it is possible that adding foliar fertilizers while forcing open plant stomata could enhance the delivery of these nutrients, I reside firmly in the skeptic camp.

This is the only remedy that I don't have an opinion on. No flowerheads, only question marks. If you enjoy talking to your plants then keep at it. It won't hurt anything and it's probably therapeutic. (I find it empowering to talk to things that won't talk back.) In terms of physiological reasons why plants might benefit from sound, it is possible that sound will close or perhaps even open stomata, but this has not been proved in any conclusive way. Some studies have shown that sound aids plant growth, but other studies have shown that sound inhibits plant growth. There is potential here, but until more research is done there are no conclusive answers as to why, how, or what sounds affect plant growth.

Vitamin B-1 🌱

This vitamin is better known as thiamin and is an important component of a sound diet for humans, but some companies have started marketing it for plants. In fact, this vitamin was shown to have a beneficial effect on plants in the 1930s! So, why aren't we using this vitamin on a regular basis? Read on.

The practice

Although vitamin B-1 is sold by itself, it is more frequently mixed with other vitamins and minerals to make biostimulants. These stimulants may be purchased as spray-on solutions but are also available as additives to hydroponic solutions or drenches to apply to soil. Vitamin B-1 is usually applied at very low concentrations, usually less than 10 parts per million.

The theory

Additions of any vitamin might work because plants cannot produce enough of these compounds for optimal growth by themselves, and they cannot find enough from the soil around them. Therefore, the theory maintains that if we simply intervene and add these vitamins to the plants, we can achieve fantastic growth. Although this theory could apply to any vitamin, vitamin B-1 is most commonly mentioned.

The real story

Plants really do use vitamin B-1. It is produced in the plants' leaves and moves through the sap to get to the plants' roots (Mozafar and Oertli 1993). Researchers have used vitamin B-1 for many years in tissue culture (basically growing plant cells in a test tube) and have found that it does encourage root growth in this kind of environment. This agrees with tests conducted on very young plants in the late 1930s (Bonner and Addicott 1937). Unfortunately, not all the tests agree with each other. Tests that look at plants larger than the youngest seedlings show that they are no larger or healthier than plants that don't have this vitamin added (Hamner 1940). It all seems to boil down to the fact that most plants are able to produce enough thiamine for themselves soon after they are able to produce leaves.

What it means to you ❀❀

Vitamin B-1 is certainly a valuable tool for those interested in growing plants in test tubes. I know many scientists who grow plants that way, and I know they appreciate thiamine. Although not much research has been done, it seems possible that vitamin B-1 might also be beneficial for rooting plants from cuttings. Using this compound on any but the smallest plants, however, is a waste of money. Larger plants (most that you buy at the store) seem to produce enough thiamine all by themselves.

Willow diffusate

Some commercially available plant hormones (auxins) can encourage root growth from cuttings. Unfortunately, not every plant responds well to auxins, and so other materials have been tried in order to elicit root growth from cuttings, some successfully and some unsuccessfully. The most infamous of these materials is willow diffusate, or willow water. Willow diffusate was first introduced by C. E. Hess in the 1950s and has been used extensively since, primarily by rose growers, some of whom swear by the stuff.

The practice

Willow diffusate is the liquid portion of a slurry of willow chips or twigs in water. One recipe for this home-brewed helper involves placing 50–100 6-inch-long willow cuttings into a gallon of water, where they sit for 4 to 6 weeks. The cuttings are then strained, and the water is used to promote root development on the cuttings of other plants. Another recipe suggests soaking sixty terminal willow stems in 4 liters of tap water for 24 hours, and yet another recommends boiling the water with the cuttings. In any case, after the stems are finished soaking, the diffusate is separated by straining the solid portions out and retaining the liquid. Cuttings of other plants can be dipped into the liquid, or the diffusate could even be used to drench the media in which the cuttings will hopefully root. If dipping the cuttings in the willow diffusate, 24 hours is commonly indicated as an appropriate length of time for them to steep in the concoction so that they can soak up the useful juices before being placed into propagation trays.

The theory

The original, overriding rationale for using willow diffusate seems akin to the old cannibal concept of eating the heart of your enemy in order to gain his courage. If a plant is easy to propagate by using stem cuttings, it stands to reason (at least to the proponents of this practice) that the plant contains substances that cause this rooting to occur. Hence, if you can somehow extract these substances and apply them to a cutting from a difficult-to-root plant, it will root more easily.

The real story

The earliest studies on this topic actually compare the rooting achieved with diffusates from easy-to-root plants to that achieved with diffusates from hard-to-root plants (Hess 1959). These original studies showed that plants treated with diffusates from easy-to-root plants were more likely to produce roots. Other, more recent, studies investigating diffusates from such plants as ivy and black locust have shown that they, too, have some ability to promote roots in other plants (Girourd and Hess 1964; Arena et al. 1997), though willow diffusate is still the most common. Perhaps the greatest users of willow diffusate are rose growers. Interestingly, roses are generally one of the easiest plants to root from stem cuttings (with a few exceptions), and were rooted through stem cuttings long before willow water or synthetic auxins were used (Bailey 1915). So when someone values willow diffusate based on their experience with roses, one wonders whether those roses might not have rooted anyway.

There is not a great deal of scientific literature that lists willow diffusate's usefulness; in fact, there is quite little. Research has actually shown that this compound inhibits the root-producing process when propagating dogwoods from very small sections of stem (Sharma and Trigiano 1999). I have tried willow diffusate myself for rooting forsythia and have found it to be much less effective than commercial rooting aids—so much less effective that applying nothing was just as good.

Although the theory behind using willow diffusate seems rather dubious at first, and my experience has led me to believe the stuff is a waste of time, some modern research supports using willow as a rooting aid. Willow is known to contain salicylic acid, better known as aspirin. Aspirin is an ethylene inhibitor. Ethylene is a plant hormone known to negatively affect cuttings, so blocking this compound could potentially encourage rooting. Indeed, salicylic acid has been shown to increase the rooting of faba bean in certain situations (Khalafalla and Hattori 2000). Unfortunately, faba beans, as well as mung beans (another plant shown to benefit from willow diffusate), seem to root with the addition of almost anything, so it is difficult to take this research as proof that willow diffusate actually works, though it is certainly a start. Much of the research that shows willow diffusate helps cuttings to develop roots uses cuttings from plants that are only a year or two old. The problem is that very young plants tend to produce roots much more readily than old plants, as demonstrated by F. E. Gardner back in 1929. Just because you were able to produce roots on cuttings taken from young plants doesn't mean you will be able to do the same thing with cuttings taken from older plants of the same type.

What it means to you ❀❀

Willow diffusate may have some value to some plants, and there are some physiological and biochemical reasons why it might work. Unfortunately, most people who try this practice on anything but easy-to-root plants wind up discouraged. Commercial rooting hormones that include the compounds indole-3-butyric acid or naphthalene-3-acetic acid are much more likely than willow diffusate to produce healthy rooted cuttings.

Putting it all together

The best thing to know about biostimulants is that you never need one. The second best thing to know is that many of the biostimulants covered in this chapter are beneficial simply because of the nutrients they contain, and although that isn't what they're sold for, there's nothing wrong with getting a little bonus. In terms of how well they do what they're supposed to— sometimes they live up to the hype, and sometimes they don't.

Rooting Plants

If there are two biostimulants you can count on, they are IBA and NAA when used to root cuttings. These compounds work, and even if they're not needed for the particular cuttings you have, they will probably still increase the number and length of roots that are produced. The only competitor that these compounds have is willow diffusate, and it really doesn't provide much competition at all once you read through the literature and try the technique yourself.

Stimulating Growth

The biostimulant with the best chance to offer anything useful for stimulating growth is, again, IBA. Using a commercial root stimulator with a low concentration of this hormone could help trees that are being transplanted by promoting root growth. This aid is not completely reliable, but has certainly been demonstrated in some situations.

Biostimulants besides IBA and NAA intended to help stimulate growth have not been particularly successful. The greatest chance of providing benefit comes from sound coupled with an application of a foliar fertilizer, though the benefit is probably from the nutrients in the fertilizer rather than the sound. Few biostimulants can reliably offer anything beyond their nutrients. When you come down to it, there just isn't much reason to believe that products such as seaweed extract and vitamin B-1 will reliably provide the fantastic results advertised.

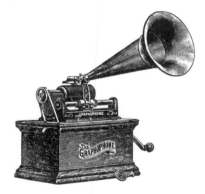

5

Insecticides

FIRST, a disclaimer. Few pesticides or other protectants in this book will have a rating of five. Why? Because few should be used unless a problem is identified. A rating of five means that the practice in question is usually beneficial, but because these products are only effective if a pest is present or a pest attack is imminent, it isn't appropriate to recommend them indiscriminately. Okay, now that we're past that, let's take a look at some pesticides.

Organic pesticides have taken on a life of their own over the past few years as people become more and more concerned about the possible effects of synthetic chemicals on humans and the environment. They often cite studies showing that synthetic pesticides are either toxic or carcinogenic to humans, dogs, or other animals. I certainly agree that many synthetic compounds we use can be toxic, carcinogenic, mutagenic, teratogenic, and more, but so can the organic pesticides we use such as rotenone and pyrethrin. In fact, rotenone is one of my least favorite pesticides because some producers seem to think that because the stuff is organic it's safe. They use it almost like water. The truth is that rotenone has been shown to be at least as toxic, if not more toxic, than most of the synthetic compounds used around the house. But rotenone is only the tip of the iceberg when talking about the potential dangers of organic pesticides. This is not to say that organic pesticides are more dangerous than synthetics. They generally aren't, but they have the potential to cause environmental problems just like synthetics do.

In 1992 Joseph Kovach, then at Cornell University, and other researchers wrote a paper titled "A Method to Measure the Environmental Impact of Pesticides." In my opinion this paper should be required reading for anyone interested in growing plants organically. In this paper Dr. Kovach looked at the relative dangers of various pesticides based on a variety of criteria, such as how toxic the pesticide is to humans and beneficial insects, and gave each pesticide a numeric value for each criterion. Higher values indicated greater danger. The numbers for each criterion could be added together to indicate a pesticide's Environmental Impact Quotient (EIQ). The higher the EIQ the more potential a pesticide has for affecting the environment. What he found was quite sobering. In general EIQ's were roughly similar between organic and synthetic pesticides. However, after taking into account the number of times a pesticide had to be applied to achieve an acceptable level of control, organic production actually had a higher potential impact on the environment. Many more applications of organic products had to be made to get the same level of control as fewer applications of synthetics. Dr. Kovach went on to show that Integrated Pest Management (IPM), which, simply put, is a method of using pesticides (usually synthetic) wisely, had the least environmental impact. I hope the conclusion is memorable: judicious use of pesticides, be they organic or synthetic, is the best way to avoid damaging the environment.

If you choose to use pesticides, you had better think long and hard about the other possible effects you could have on the environment. The difference between synthetic and organic pesticides and their home-brewed counterparts is that the commercial products include information on how to use them safely. You get no such instructions from do-it-yourself guides. Most of the commercial pesticides today are quite effective and relatively safe if the labeled instructions are closely followed and good common sense is used.

Many homemade brews can affect the life of an insect on your favorite plant. Most are actually somewhat effective against insect pests, and at least a few have been used for many years. Some are not true insecticides at all but rather repellents that deter insects instead of killing them. Deterrents are a useful way to stop insect damage, but be careful to cover everything you want to protect. Otherwise you will be saving one plant just to see the insects move to another, untreated plant.

Citrus peel

Citrus peels have been suggested as a cure for ants and as a source of natural insecticidal compounds. E. A. Back and C. E. Pemberton showed in 1915 that the oils from citrus fruits can affect insects, but those oils haven't really been used for insect control until relatively recently. The important event in the rediscovery of citrus peels was when entomologist Craig Sheppard recognized the effects of an orange hand soap on ants (Olkowski et al. 1991), and now this natural product is found in both commercial insecticidal sprays and in home-brewed remedies.

The practice

To control ants, do-it-yourself guides sometimes recommend placing citrus peels over an ant mound. They may further recommend a natural insecticidal spray made of water mixed with citrus peel. A recipe for this type of spray typically includes mixing the peel of one or two oranges (or limes) with 2–4 cups of boiling water. This mixture is allowed to steep for up to 24 hours. Some recommendations include adding a drop or two of soap, usually dish soap, to the mixture either before or after the citrus peel is steeped.

The theory

Citrus peels are thought to contain insecticidal compounds, most notably limonene (more properly called d-limonene), that can be easily extracted and applied to control insects.

The real story

Limonene is known to be toxic to insects and has some effect on mites as well (Ibrahim et al. 2001; Lee et al. 1997). There are currently a number of commercial insecticides that contain limonene and are considered organic. Limonene has one major drawback: it tends to damage plants (Ibrahim et al. 2001). Any application of citrus peels or concoctions made from citrus need to be checked out on plants that you are willing to damage before they are tried on your high-value plants.

Having a natural curiosity about anything to do with repelling ants—a curiosity that anyone who has lived around fire ants will probably share—I decided to take a look at using orange peels to get rid of ant mounds. Since I did not have access to fire ants here in chilly Minnesota I tested oranges on their smaller northern cousins. I applied either orange peels or orange peel puree in large quantities to ant mounds. The results were amazingly unconvincing. The ants simply did not care, in either case, that I had surrounded their homes with what was supposed to be a toxic substance. In the case of the puree, I actually formed a barrier around their entrance hole to force them to contact the stuff. The ants walked right over it and then moved the crusted pieces after they dried out a few days later.

Based on my results, the biggest potential problem with making home remedies out of citrus peel does not seem to have anything to do with potential damage to your plant from the mixture, though this is certainly a major consideration. Rather, it has to do with the concentration of limonene in the citrus peel. Commercial products are usually applied with anywhere from 1 percent to 6 percent limonene in the spray solution. Although the recipes above would certainly get some limonene onto the insect, it is unlikely that these sprays would have a concentration even remotely close to the concentration of limonene present in commercial sprays. Because limonene is an oily substance, soap would have to be added to mix the limonene with the water. The addition of soap, which may well damage plants, makes a mixture that is probably worth avoiding.

What it means to you ✿✿✿

Based on the research conducted by other scientists I see no reason to believe that commercial formulations of limonene shouldn't be effective against many insects, though these formulations are probably not appropriate for use on plants. Citrus peels in homemade concoctions, on the other hand, don't seem like a valuable remedy for insect problems.

If you still want to try citrus peels in a homebrew, despite the information offered here, the best recipe is one that recommends adding the grated peels of at least two oranges per cup of boiling water, with 1 or 2 tablespoons of soap added to the water prior to adding the orange peel, and soaking the peels for a full 24 hours before using the spray. This recipe is more likely to be effective because it should allow more of the limonene to get into the spray and because it includes soap, which can be quite an effective insecticide in and of itself. As with most of these homemade remedies, if you insist on using it, remember to test it on plants you are willing to lose before you spray it on anything that you value.

Dish soap

Dish soaps, along with other types of soap, are common ingredients in home-brewed concoctions recommended by garden gurus for getting rid of injurious soft bodied insects such as scale and aphids. Some soaps have also been recommended as antifungal agents. Soap has been used as a method for controlling insects since the 1700s. In fact, in the early 1800s a recipe for urine and soap was all the rage for getting rid of aphids on melons (yum-yum) (Lodeman 1906). Soap's ability to ward off diseases such as powdery mildew, a common fungus attacking many plants, is less known. Surprisingly, despite references in old literature to the use of soaps for insects, little mention is ever made of using soaps to control fungi.

The practice

Dish soap is mixed with water and applied to the plant via a sprayer. Many different concentrations are recommended depending upon the source, but typically about 1–4 tablespoons are recommended per gallon of water. Oil, such as vegetable oil, is often also added at about the same concentration.

The theory

Dish soap is supposed to "clean up" soft-bodied insects by washing off the wax cuticle that surrounds the body of all insects. Once the wax cuticle is removed, the insect is unable to retain its body moisture and will dry up and die. Hard-bodied insects, such as beetles, have a shell that is more impervious to water than that of soft-bodied insects, so hard-bodied insects are less prone to being killed by applications of soap. For fungal diseases, which are spread by spores, soaps supposedly disturb the integrity of the membrane surrounding the spore, causing it to split open and die.

Commercially produced insecticidal soaps can be purchased at most garden centers. (Soaps created specifically for harmful fungi are rarely seen on garden center shelves.) These soaps, however, are expensive compared to everyday dish soaps. Most garden gurus believe that dish soap should be able to do the same job as insecticidal soap for a fraction of the cost.

The real story

When researchers tested insecticidal soap and dish soap in a side-by-side comparison of their ability to control whiteflies on tomatoes, both reduced whitefly populations. In fact, the dish soap actually did a better job than the insecticidal soap. Unfortunately, the dish soap also caused significant damage to the tomato plants. The research showed an interesting but not unexpected trend. The greater the effect that a particular soap had on the whitefly population, the greater the effect that soap had on the plant (Sclar et al. 1999).

How can soaps injure plants? Plants have wax cuticles, just like insects have, and that cuticle can be removed with the application of soap, just like an insect's can. Removal of wax doesn't kill the plant outright, as it might an insect, but it does allow water to be lost from leaves. The water loss leads to leaf scorch and leaf drop and can weaken the plant, eventually resulting in death. Different soaps have different abilities to remove the plant's natural cuticle, and insecticidal soaps have been specially formulated to try to preserve the plant's wax cuticle while regular dish soap has not. Insecticidal soaps are made with the plant's safety in mind. Therefore, these products may sacrifice some effectiveness in killing the pest population for the benefit of not killing plants outright. Nonetheless, most research shows that with proper application methods insecticidal soaps are very effective on aphids and other pests (Fournier and Brodeur 2000; Braman and Latimer 2002).

Some dish soaps have done quite well in controlling powdery mildew. In a study conducted by M. T. Mmbaga and H. Sheng (2002), Palmolive was quite effective for controlling this disease on dogwood, as was Ajax and Equate. Generally, when insecticidal soaps were tested side by side against dish soaps in their ability to control powdery mildew, the dish soaps performed better. Unfortunately, Palmolive was found to be quite damaging to the plant material tested.

What it means to you ❀❀❀

Commercially available insecticidal soaps are a great idea, and these products are not used nearly enough. They are safe for the environment, generally quite effective on the pests that they are supposed to target, and usually safe for the plant. There are few soaps sold for the control of fungi in plants, so using them for this purpose is not a great idea unless you can find a soap specifically labeled for it.

Dish soaps can be an adequate replacement for commercially produced insecticidal soaps, and in fact may even kill pests more effectively than commercial insecticidal soaps. But without first testing them on plants you are willing to damage or even kill, you are playing Russian roulette. The wrong amount of soap will either be ineffective or hurt your plant. If you are willing to experiment (and damage some plants in the process!), then dish soaps are a good idea, but for the everyday gardener, it's probably a better idea to put up the extra $2 and buy some soap formulated specifically to clean off the insects. Finally, before you apply any soap, be sure you are not applying antibacterial soaps, as these tend to be more harmful to plants.

Forsyth's composition

Some pesticides that were used years ago have a place in our current pesticide arsenal. Bordeaux mixture, pyrethrum, and rotenone are all available commercially for pest control today, though they were discovered long ago. The pesticides used most frequently in past times, however, tended to be unreliable. One well-known insecticide of the late 18th and early 19th centuries was Forsyth's composition. This pesticide is very representative of the type of pesticides that typically found their way onto crops during this era.

William Forsyth is a name that is respected by gardeners and plantaholics across the globe. He was King George III's gardener and was renowned as one of the greatest plantsmen of his time. The genus *Forsythia* is named after this pillar of the plant world. As a great plantsman, Forsyth often had the need to apply pesticides to his plants to keep them healthy. A great plantsman he was; a great chemist he was not.

The practice

Forsyth's composition, which he recommended in 1791, consisted of 1 bushel of cow dung, ½ bushel of lime rubbish from old buildings, ½ bushel of wood ash, and 1/16 bushel of river sand. This mixture was finely sifted and mixed with urine or soapy water until it was the consistency of paint. At this point it could be applied to the plant. After application, he recommended that a dry powder containing wood ash and bone ash at a ratio of

6:1 should be dusted over it. This compound corrected problems with insect infestations and was also considered especially good for covering tree wounds (Lodeman 1906; Mercer 1979).

The theory

Science as a practice really hasn't been around for that long. Nowhere is that more obvious than the reasoning behind Forsyth's composition. Compounds used during Forsyth's time were considered desirable if they had great "strength." A compound's strength was based primarily on its odor; the more disagreeable the odor, the more likely that the compound would be effective. Common high-strength compounds used for controlling insects included pigeon dung, urine, vinegar, and others too horrendous to name.

The real story

Some ingredients Forsyth named do have value. Lime, for example, is known to have some effect on insects and was commonly used years after Forsyth's composition was recommended (Weed 1915). To my knowledge the primary ingredient, cow dung, has never been shown to have any effect on insects, except perhaps dung beetles, so it is hard to surmise what the cow dung offered to the mixture besides consistency and smell. Wood ash and river sand, likewise, would probably offer little in the way of insecticidal properties but were probably used primarily to offer consistency and texture. The urine and especially the soap suds could well have offered some insecticidal properties, much like today's insecticidal soaps.

What it means to you ❀❀

Forsyth's composition is one of those old homemade recipes that has not found favor in our modern age, and for good reason. I have never found this mixture particularly appealing as an insect control agent, and I don't think I ever will. Most of the insecticides and fungicides developed around that time that were actually useful can still be purchased today. If they can't, you can safely assume they probably weren't particularly useful.

Garlic

Eating garlic is a quick and easy way to prepare for a dinner party at which there will be no one you particularly care to talk to. We are all aware of garlic's repellent qualities as it applies to humans, but might these properties apply to insects, too? Unlike so many other homemade insect repellents in do-it-yourself guides, garlic is not easily found in old gardening and insect-control literature. In fact, garlic has really only been suggested for home-made insect-control mixtures over the last 30 years or so.

The practice

Many different forms of garlic are available, including commercially prepared garlic sprays, garlic extract, garlic oils, and, of course, garlic cloves. Commercially prepared garlic sprays should be applied as per the instructions on the container. The home-brewed remedy fanatic has a number of recipes for garlic oils and garlic extracts to choose from. Perhaps the best recipe comes from a scientific article written by H. M. Flint and his colleagues in 1995 about their use of a garlic extract to control whiteflies. A homeowner could easily make this recipe for insect control. It includes 125 grams (about 4.4 ounces) of garlic extract mixed with a small amount of soap (a few drops of insecticidal soap would work) and 1 liter (a little more than 1 quart) of water. This mixture is then blended and strained through 2 pieces of cheesecloth. The resulting mixture is diluted with water to 10 percent of its original concentration. Other recipes involve mixing one garlic bulb with 2 cups of water, blending thoroughly, straining, and mixing the liquid with a gallon of water for spraying. Another recommendation suggests mixing garlic with other potential insecticides, such as orange peel, for increased benefit.

The theory

Garlic contains a number of compounds, including diallyl disulfide and diallyl trisulfide, that are supposed to be repellent or deadly to insects.

The real story

Although garlic sprays weren't used on insects until the 1970s, as early as the 1950s garlic extracts were known to affect ticks (Catar 1954). Garlic was first reported as an insecticidal compound in 1970 when S. V. Amonkar and E. L. Reeves found that it could be used at very low concentrations to poison mosquito larvae.

Research has shown that a number of insects are repelled by garlic sprays, including whiteflies, aphids, and beetles (Flint et al. 1995; Hori

1996; Huang et al. 2000). Research has also shown that, while sprays may be toxic to insects, the repellency of the garlic means that insects rarely hang around long enough for death to occur. Some good news for the do-it-yourselfer is that Flint's garlic extract recipe seems to be more effective than commercially purchased garlic oil preparations. Unfortunately, the smell of the homemade applications tends to last for about a week, which is considerably longer than commercial formulations. This probably means the homemade formula will repel insects for longer than the commercial formula, but it also means your nose will be assailed by this pungent aroma for longer. Getting good coverage of plants with the spray is extremely important because if a leaf is missed, that is where insects will congregate.

What it means to you ❀❀❀❀

Garlic works, plain and simple. Plants will smell like garlic for a considerable time after it is applied, but if you are opposed to using commercial insecticides this is a great choice. One important observation: for this spray to be effective, good coverage is essential—try not to miss a leaf. Repellents for insects are somewhat controversial because of their fundamental trait (repelling an insect versus killing it); they tend to shift an insect population rather than wiping it out. If a portion of the plant is not sprayed, the insect pest will decimate that portion. Likewise, if a portion of your garden is treated but the rest of the garden is left unsprayed, then the insects will simply move to the untreated plants. Dish soap makes garlic sprays more effective, but it will also make them more dangerous to your plants. As always, if you're convinced that you want to use garlic, be sure to test it on plants that you can afford to lose.

One final note. I have seen garlic recommended for flea control on dogs, but if your dog likes to be patted and if you or your friends don't like their hands to smell like garlic, this is probably not a good idea.

Hellebore 🌱

Hellebore is a classic insecticide that has not found much favor in today's pest-control recommendations, though it was certainly effective for its time. In some organic pest-control books information on hellebore can still be found, but by and large its use went out of favor in the 1920s and 1930s.

This insecticide is not derived from true hellebore (the genus *Helleborus*) but rather from two unrelated plants, American hellebore and white hellebore (*Veratrum viride* and *V. album*). These plants are extremely toxic and should not be eaten, or even touched, if it can be avoided.

The practice

Hellebore recipes are quite varied. Typically 1 ounce of dried, powdered roots are applied directly to the plant. If a spray-on solution is used, hellebore concentrations can range from 1 ounce of hellebore mixed with 3 gallons of water to 2 ounces of hellebore for every 1 gallon of water (Lodeman 1906; Metcalf and Flint 1939).

The theory

Hellebore has long been known as a toxic plant. This plant is supposed to act as a stomach poison so that when eaten it will affect the insect's stomach and result in death.

The real story

Modern research has paid little attention to this old-time botanical insecticide, and few studies investigate how well this insecticide works when compared to modern insecticides. Old literature indicates that it was about ⅓ as toxic to insects as lead arsenate, another old pesticide that is a little too toxic to humans and other mammals for modern use (Metcalf and Flint 1939). Hellebore contains toxic alkaloids that are the source of the plant's toxicity.

What it means to you ❀❀

Hellebore is a very poisonous plant and should be treated as such. Modern insecticides tend to be more effective on insects and less toxic to humans than concoctions made with *Veratrum*, making it difficult to suggest this plant as a pest-control compound.

Hot peppers for unwanted guests

Eating hot peppers hurts, no two ways about it. Can the heat we feel when eating hot peppers be used to help control insects? Hot peppers, specifically cayenne peppers, have been used in concoctions for some time. In his popular book, *New American Orchardist*, published in 1833, Dr. William Kenrick recommended syringing a cayenne pepper solution onto plants to kill aphids. Since then many people, especially organic gardeners, have tried using hot peppers for pests.

Today we know that hot peppers contain a compound called capsaicin, which makes our tongues feel like fire and is supposedly very good at warding off pests. After all, if it works on us it makes sense that this chemical should work on everything from insects to deer and rodents—right?

The practice

Capsaicin can be purchased in a more-or-less pure form in deer and insect repellents and is often referred to as "hot pepper sauce" or something similar. This chemical can also be purchased as a natural component of hot sauces used to flavor food, Tabasco being the most common. Chapter 8 discusses capsaicin for use against deer and rodents; the information here concerns its use in controlling insects.

For commercial insecticides utilizing capsaicin, label recommendation should be followed, but for home-brewed remedies, one of many hot sauces may be added to water at a concentration of a few tablespoons per gallon of water. A tablespoon or two of dish soap is often added to this mixture as well, which can then be sprayed on plants to control insects. People who really want to put together a concoction from the ground up should mix ½–2 cups of the hottest peppers you can find with 2 cups of water, mix the peppers and water in a blender, and strain the resulting liquid. The strained liquid can then be applied directly to plants with or without 1 or 2 tablespoons of dish soap. If you decide to mix your own hot pepper spray, be sure to use gloves. Capsaicin can be painful if too much gets on your hands.

The theory

If it tastes hot to us then, the gurus believe, it should taste hot to insects and other pests.

The real story

Capsaicin has been shown to deter insects, though not necessarily to kill them (Cowles et al. 1989). In some studies, commercial formulations of capsaicin were shown to repel insects, including mites and whiteflies, for up to 2 months (Madanlar et al. 2002). These studies were conducted in a greenhouse, and it is unlikely this spray would last as long in an outdoor garden. However, it is still quite a remarkable achievement. As with other repellents, if capsaicin is only applied to one group of plants in a garden and not another, insects will simply concentrate on the untreated plants. Likewise, if a plant is only sprayed over a small portion of its leaves, only those leaves that have been sprayed will be protected from insects. With all this spraying going on, it is good to know that the danger of capsaicin to foliage has been investigated on tender herbs, and it does not appear to damage plants (Cloyd and Cycholl 2002). Any additional ingredients, such as a soap, added to the spray could change that. Remember that pepper spray is used as a human deterrent and that a homemade pepper recipe could adversely affect someone accidentally sprayed with it.

What it means to you 🌻🌻🌻🌻

Capsaicin is likely to help control insect infestations, especially mite and whitefly infestations. Because capsaicin is a repellent rather than a poison, don't expect to wipe out pests overnight. Homemade hot pepper sprays will not be as effective as store-bought pepper spays because commercial producers put more time and effort into making sprays than homeowners will. Most of these commercial sprays include additives that allow the capsaicin to stay on the plant for a long period of time; homemade remedies will not last as long and will need to be reapplied often. It is possible that homemade hot pepper sprays, which usually include dish soap, will be somewhat damaging to plants and may burn them.

Nematodes 🌱

Little worms too small to see without a microscope, wriggling around and eating a living body from the inside out, slowly creating a breeding ground for themselves inside their host. Sound like a bad horror movie? It's not. Small worms, called nematodes, can be purchased and applied to your soil. These worms enter the body of the insect and eat it from the inside out over a period of a few days or weeks, providing a grizzly weapon in the war against garden pests.

You can buy two types of nematodes for your garden, the genera *Stein-*

ernema and *Heterorhabditis*. These little guys would obviously make a great movie. But will they do as well in a garden as they would at the box office?

The practice

Nematodes are purchased by the millions and applied at concentrations of anywhere from one million to ten million nematodes per 1000 square feet. The nematodes usually come mixed in dry clay, which is added to water to produce a spray that will disseminate these little critters. They are usually recommended for the control of soil-dwelling pests such as grubs, crickets, and some caterpillars.

The theory

Since nematodes need to eat insects to live and reproduce, it stands to reason that if enough are introduced to an area they will eat all the "bad" insects.

The real story

It has been known for years that some nematodes can infect and kill insects, but not until 1931 did R. W. Glaser manage to grow nematodes without an insect host. This was an extremely important event in the use of these critters as an insect control because it is nearly impossible to collect enough nematodes to sell if you only harvest them from dead insects. In 1934 the first attempts were made at introducing nematodes to an area to control an insect. *Steinernema glaseri* (then called *Neoaplectana glaseri*) was used against the Japanese beetle (Steinhaus 1949). This study demonstrated something all users of nematodes need to know, which is, in a nutshell, that nematodes are somewhat fickle. In fact, the number of Japanese beetles infected with this nematode ranged from 0.3 to 81.5 percent, depending on environmental conditions. The researchers studying these nematodes found that they function best in warm soil—over 60 degrees Fahrenheit (15.5 degrees Celsius)—that is moist but not flooded. Additionally, they prefer not to be applied to cultivated soil and like a large number of host insects to be readily available (Girth et al. 1940). You could think of it as providing your nematode guests with a nice restaurant: plenty of food, not too much air conditioning, an attentive busboy to keep the water glass filled, and beautiful green surroundings.

As long as environmental conditions are conducive to their activity, you can count on nematodes, regardless of species, to be effective against most insects that spend a portion of their life cycle in the soil, including such pests as the plum curculio, Japanese beetles, and crickets (Shapiro et al. 2004; Girth et al. 1940; Wang et al. 1994). The most common nematode for sale today is *Steinernema carpocapsae*, which has achieved popularity because it can affect many different types of insects and is a voracious feeder.

Pesticides are detrimental to many biological control agents. Nematodes tend to fare much better than most people expect when subjected to many common pesticides, making them extremely attractive to those who would like the option of using chemicals if necessary (deNardo and Grewal 2003; Gupta and Siddiqui 1999; Rovesti et al. 1990).

One of the biggest drawbacks to nematodes is their cost and storage considerations. Nematodes often cost ten times or more what it would cost to apply a pesticide. Since nematodes can reproduce themselves, however, they often last a lot longer than pesticides and may hang around for 5 years or longer if insects are available for them to feed on (Girth et al. 1940). Because they are living creatures, nematodes cannot be stored for long and most businesses that sell them recommend applying them immediately or, if that is not possible, storing them for less than a week in a refrigerator.

What it means to you ❀❀❀❀

Nematodes are very effective killers of soil-dwelling insects. They will not wipe out pest populations and leave their children with nothing to eat, but if environmental conditions are correct, with warm soil and high moisture, they can make quite a dent in a group of soil-dwelling pests. Since the pests that nematodes target are in the soil, the fact that nematodes kill insects slowly shouldn't overly concern you. After all, you won't have to witness the suffering grubs that your nematodes feast on. Be aware that nematodes are somewhat expensive, and they should be used promptly after receipt from the supply company.

Predators and parasites 🐛

You can buy all kinds of insect predators and parasites to control the harmful insects in your garden. The web is simply full of sources of these magnificent little beasties. The advertisements usually say that adding predatory insects achieves a natural predator-prey or parasite-prey balance in situations that are unbalanced. This may be true, but if you think you should apply predatory insects, you should first be aware of some of their characteristics.

The practice

Insect predators and parasites are purchased and then released into a garden, greenhouse, or field. They are rarely used with any sort of synthetic, or even organic, insecticide, as those compounds tend to kill beneficial insects even more effectively than they kill pest insects.

The theory

Predators or parasites should control unwanted insects by eating or parasitizing them, eliminating the need for pesticide applications.

The real story

To understand insect predators and parasites you need to divide them into groups; not all predators and parasites are created equal. They differ in their ability to eat large numbers of pest insects, in their preferred prey range, and in their desire and ability to migrate out of the location where they were originally placed. Never underestimate the ability of insects to find food, and if that means leaving your garden, they'll do it.

Cost and survival are the biggest problems with natural predators and parasites. These beneficial insects do not come cheaply, and they do not like to be mailed across the entire United States. Usually everything works out fine, but too much heat or cold during shipping can have quite an effect on the survival of your insects.

Lady beetles. Lady beetles are extremely effective predators. Various types of lady beetles can be purchased, but two species are more common than others: *Hippodamia convergens* and *Cryptolaemus montrouzieri*. *Cryptolaemus* is more commonly known as the mealybug destroyer and really lives up to its name. Many, if not most, botanical gardens in the United States release this insect in their conservatories to control mealybugs as well as aphids and scale to a lesser extent. These insects are most appropriate for greenhouses and other enclosed spaces, but they could be, and often are, released into gardens. The biggest problem with a release of *Cryptolaemus* is that if insect populations are low, this critter is just going to fly off to find prey elsewhere. The other lady beetle you are likely to encounter though, *Hippodamia convergens*, also known as the convergent lady beetle, is even worse at sticking around than *Cryptolaemus*. Only by understanding how these beetles are collected can we understand why they are such transient guests.

Convergent lady beetles sold through the mail are usually collected over the winter. This is important because lady beetles like to spend the winter snuggled up into the bark of a tree or some other semi-enclosed area. When the winter ends the lady beetles, who usually spend the season in close proximity to each other, like to migrate far from the location where they spent the winter (Rankin and Rankin 1980), probably so they don't have to compete with their former bunkmates for food. When you get your box of lady beetles fresh from the cooler (that's where they have to be stored after they're collected) they are all ready to disperse to find prey. If they are released in your garden expect them to disperse from your garden, with only a few lady beetles choosing to stick around. All this said, convergent lady beetles are excellent predators, and if they decide to hang around, which is unlikely, they are a very welcome addition to almost any garden.

Preying mantis. The preying mantis is a fantastically beautiful insect that is a joy to see in your garden, but it is not particularly effective at controlling pests. Mantises are inefficient predators because they tend not to congregate in large numbers.

Lacewings. Lacewings are a little-known and underutilized predator. Lacewing adults are very pretty with green bodies and gossamer wings, but it is their ugly larvae that are effective at killing pests. When you purchase lacewings you usually get eggs, though sometimes you may receive adults. Eggs are generally preferred because the larvae that hatch from them cannot migrate like the adults. Lacewing larvae look like tiny alligators and are incredibly voracious, eating mites, aphids, whiteflies, and others. I have even seen these guys become cannibals if there is not enough other food available.

Minute pirate bug. I really shouldn't play favorites, but sometimes I just can't help it. The minute pirate bug is my favorite predatory insect, attacking thrips, mites, aphids, young caterpillars, and many other pests. This is a small insect that has proved itself time and time again as a wonderful predator with a wide variety of tastes, but it is best known as a spider mite killer and is effective against these little guys as well as against thrips (Wilson et al. 1991; Higgins 1992). One nice aspect of the minute pirate bug is that, while it can fly, it tends to stay around your garden as long as something is available for it to eat. Don't think that this means you can't release this predator if you don't see any pests, though. The minute pirate bug also feeds on pollen, so if you have some flowers blooming and want to release this insect to defend against something you suspect could pop up in the near future, then go for it.

Big eyed bug. The big eyed bug is very similar to the minute pirate bug in size. When I lived in Georgia I would sometimes see this insect on dandelions, feeding on the pollen. One day I took one off a dandelion to get a closer look, and it bit me right on the webbing of my fingers. It didn't hurt much, but it is remarkable that an insect only about $\frac{1}{10}$ of an inch long or less can give you a nip that you can feel at all. The big eyed bug is very similar to the minute pirate bug in its prey and abilities.

Parasitic wasps. By far the most common parasitic wasp on the market is the greenhouse whitefly parasite, *Encarsia formosa*. This tiny wasp lays eggs inside immature whiteflies, which hatch and eat the young whitefly from the inside out. The wasps are incredibly effective in enclosed spaces, such as greenhouses, but are less effective outside because wind will blow them away from the area where you released them. The biggest problem with these insects is their host range. They will control whiteflies, but nothing else. The aphid parasite *Aphidius colemani* is effective against many aphids, but has the same problems as the whitefly parasite: it will only attack aphids and can blow to other areas if it is released out of doors.

A somewhat less commonly available group of parasites are wasps in the genus *Trichogramma*. These wasps attack the eggs of various moths, killing the pests before they can ever turn into caterpillars. *Trichogramma* wasps usually arrive at your doorstep in moth eggs that are ready to be spread around infested plants. Wasps hatch out of the eggs, often two or three per egg, and then attack the eggs of other moths. *Trichogramma* wasps have a reputation for being effective at controlling harmful caterpillars in large scale cropping operations, such as cotton fields. Their usefulness on a smaller scale, such as a garden, is a little less certain because they are extremely small (they live in moth eggs after all); they have the same propensity as other parasitic wasps have to be blown away. For this reason, they and other parasitic wasps are usually best applied numerous times over the course of a year.

Predatory mites. Predatory mites, such as *Phytoseiulus persimilis* and *Metaseiulus occidentalis*, are effective against other mites such as the two-spotted spider mite and European red mite. Although certain predatory mites can affect insects, such as thrips, the minute pirate bug or big eyed bug are probably better choices. These mites are so tiny that you can't see them unless you're really looking for them, and even then a hand lens is useful. There is no doubt that these are extremely valuable predators, but make sure mites are indeed the problem before you send in predatory mites. I tend to prefer the minute pirate bug simply because I usually have more problems than just spider mites on my plants.

What it means to you ✿✿✿✿✿

Natural predators are great. They get a rating of five because even if you choose the wrong predator and apply it at the wrong time, you're not going to hurt anything and may even have a beneficial impact despite yourself. The same cannot be said for most commercial insecticides.

The biggest problem with applying beneficial insects and mites is that these guys are set up to fail. Most of us tend to wait until a pest population is beyond repair before we release them, making it impossible for the fantastic little beasts to provide the sort of pest control we would like to see. Beneficial predators and parasites need to be released before a pest population goes gangbusters, not after. Finally, with few exceptions, releasing beneficial predators and parasites is not compatible with the use of pesticides.

Tobacco ☘

Tobacco has a long history with humans, both as an intoxicant and as an insecticide. The first mention of using tobacco to kill insects dates back to the late 17th century, when Jean de la Quintinye, gardener to King Louis XIV, published his book *Instruction pour les Jardins Fruitiers et Potages* (1690). If you have ever paged through gardening books published before 1930 to find remedies for insect problems then you have probably already established that tobacco was one of the best-loved insecticides. An old USDA manuscript by N. E. McIndoo and R. C. Roark titled *A Bibliography of Nico-*

tine (1936) is a 345-page list of papers and books on the subject that have been published over the last few centuries.

Concoctions including tobacco are considered the gold standard of insect control for the home-remedy connoisseur. Tobacco has developed a very effective set of defensive compounds for itself over the years that are very effective at poisoning the herbivores that try to feed on it. Humans, seeing how effective tobacco was at poisoning these herbivores, decided quite naturally to use tobacco as an effective way to slowly poison themselves. Who knew that it would work so well? But regardless of what we do to ourselves, is tobacco a useful way to control insects on garden plants?

The practice

The most common way to apply tobacco to plants is to soak tobacco leaves, chewing tobacco, or some other tobacco product in hot water. The amount of tobacco to add varies widely between recipes, but usually anywhere from 1 tablespoon to a handful per gallon of water is used. After the tobacco has soaked for a certain length of time, somewhere between an hour and a day, the water is filtered off and applied to the plants, often with some other additive, such as a tablespoon of dish soap.

If you want to try a nicotine insecticide brewed the old fashioned way, and you have access to fresh tobacco, Clarence Weed in his book *Insects and Insecticides* (1915) recommended steeping 5 pounds of tobacco stems in 3 gallons of water for 3 hours then straining the tobacco stems off and diluting the resulting mixture with enough water to make 7 gallons of spray.

The theory

Tobacco seems to be effective at controlling people, so why not insects? Why not indeed. The same ingredient that humans find so addictive, nicotine, is a very potent nerve toxin that certainly has the potential to affect insects.

The real story

As any smoker can tell you, tobacco contains a stimulant. That stimulant is nicotine, and tobacco contains anywhere from 2 to 14 percent of this compound in its leaves, depending on the type of tobacco (Metcalf and Metcalf 1993). Basically, a stimulant causes nerve cells to fire. If you can't stop the nerve cells from firing, you start twitching and eventually die. Nicotine causes death in humans if applied at a high enough concentration; fortunately, insects require much lower concentrations to bring about their demise. Black Leaf 40 is an insecticide, now off the market, that contained nicotine (40 percent nicotine—hence the name) and was very effective on a wide variety of pests. Homemade concoctions will not be as effective as this former commercial insecticide, but they can still do quite a number on insects.

Though homemade mixtures that use tobacco are likely to work, getting the right amount of tobacco into the mix is a difficult task. Chewing tobacco is available in a wide variety of styles, which are likely to release their insecticidal compound into a home-brewed concoction differently. More finely ground tobacco should deliver more nicotine to the solution than coarsely ground types. You could get quite a range of control from home-brewed insecticides from one batch to the next if you're not careful about buying the same type of chewing tobacco every time.

Although tobacco may be our valuable ally, it can also be a terrible enemy. Chewing tobacco, because it comes from the tobacco plant, may have tobacco mosaic virus in it. This is a particularly deadly disease for certain plants, so concoctions using tobacco should never be used around ornamental tobacco, geraniums, tomatoes, potatoes, peppers, and other plants susceptible to this disease.

What it means to you ❀❀❀

Nicotine is an effective insecticide and homemade concoctions that include chaw are likely to be effective. There are a huge number of concoctions that include various amounts of tobacco. If you decide to try chewing tobacco, experiment a little bit to figure out how much of your certain type (there are many types of chewing tobaccos) you need to add to water to make a concoction that is effective on insects. Remember that the old sprays used almost a pound of tobacco per gallon of water, which is much more concentrated that the garden gurus recommend and could prove to be quite expensive and dangerous. That is a lot of snuff tins.

Remember also that the chaw you use may be host to the tobacco mosaic virus, so be careful what you treat. Also be careful if you have added any dish soap to your homemade concoction, as including it increases the likelihood that you will damage the plants. With all these caveats about using chewing tobacco wouldn't it be easier to just go out and buy some insecticidal soap?

Putting it all together

If you're willing to experiment and risk damaging a few plants, you may want to try some homebrews to help rid yourself of insect problems. Commercial pesticides do tend to be more effective than these products, but they may carry with them a higher degree of toxicity or, at least, the perception of higher toxicity. Be sure to very carefully read the label of any commercial insecticide that you decide to use, and follow the application instructions.

To control soft bodied insects and mites

Most of the control measures that rid your plants of aphids also take care of other pests, including mealy bugs, mites, and, to a lesser extent, scale. My favorite choices for controlling these critters are natural enemies, primarily the minute pirate bug and the big eyed bug. These natural enemies won't decimate pest populations quickly, though. Those who want the kill-'em-fast method should consider the many homemade and commercial options.

The most appropriate home remedy to try right away is the hose-off method. This method involves nothing more than aiming a stream of water at a population of soft bodied insects to knock them off a plant. This method works very well when you have insects on a small number of plants. The second method to try is a simple mix of soap and water. After all, most of the home-brewed remedies listed above include at least some soap, and there is no point mixing in extra stuff that you don't have to and that might make your spray more dangerous to plants. If soap doesn't work garlic, hot peppers, and tobacco are three additional ingredients that could make your soapy water more effective.

If you want to use commercial insecticides, first try insecticidal soap. If this isn't effective enough and you want to go with the big guns, take a close look at acephate, permethrin, and imidacloprid (except for use against mites). Useful organic products include oils, pyrethrin, and neem. Commercial insecticides, whether synthetic or organic, usually work, but many of them kill beneficial insects. As a result you will often need to apply more insecticides later in the season to kill the pests that your beneficial insects would have killed had you not applied the first insecticide. A vicious cycle ensues, which leads to this advice: don't apply insecticides unless you have to, and if you do have to, strongly consider soaps and oils, as these tend to be less harmful to beneficial insects.

For beetles and caterpillars

Beetles and caterpillars are more difficult to control than soft bodied insects because they have an exoskeleton that is thicker and more resistant to damage. Soaps may still be effective on these insects, but the concentration usually has to be increased to a level such that plant injury is unavoidable. Adding hot peppers, garlic, or tobacco can help the efficacy of these sprays through their repellency as well as their toxicity, but they could still negatively impact the plants you are treating. My first choice of insecticide for beetles and caterpillars is *Bacillus thuringiensis* (B.t.). This naturally occurring pesticide is a stomach toxin, and it kills insects slowly, though it stops feeding almost immediately. B.t. is very specific for the type of insects that it kills, so if you purchase one type to kill caterpillars, do not expect it to kill beetles, and vice versa. One type of B.t. will kill various types of flies, most notably mosquitoes.

If you are looking for fast-working synthetic chemicals, many are available, but first consider carbaryl and permethrin. Both of these compounds, however, are extremely hard on beneficial insects, especially lady beetles. If you do feel that you need to use them, it is best to confine their use to as small an area as possible to reduce collateral effects.

For soil-dwelling insects

Insects that live in the soil are notoriously hard to control because they have a layer of soil above them that can block the effect of anything you spray. Nematodes are my first choice for controlling soil pests such as grubs. They do not provide 100 percent control, but they can greatly reduce a population, especially under warm, moist conditions. Pesticides for controlling grubs include the synthetic insecticides imidacloprid and carbaryl, as well as the organic insecticide *Bacillus popilliae*, better known as milky spore disease. However, milky spore disease is only effective with Japanese beetle larvae.

For wasps and hornets

No home-brewed remedy does a particularly effective job against wasps and hornets. Not that the homebrews won't kill them; you just want to kill them fast enough so that you don't get stung. Most commercial insecticides intended for use on these pests work extremely rapidly, but most are also synthetic. An exception to this is mint oil, which is supposed to knock down insects relatively rapidly.

For ants

As with many other insects, soapy water will kill ants, and tobacco or garlic will make it more toxic. The organic spray limonene is quite effective on ants but is not safe for plants. Most of the synthetic sprays for ants, such as permethrin, are also effective. Diatomaceous earth is another organic pesticide that can be spread to block the ants' movement.

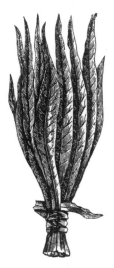

6

Fungicides and Other Disease-Control Agents

MANY HOMEMADE concoctions are supposed to control diseases; some have been tested extensively in a scientific way, but most haven't. In fact, most of the home-brewed disease controls haven't been studied. In order to rectify this problem, we conducted a test to examine how well a few of the more-common homemade disease controls fared against two of the problems that many typical gardeners are worried about, powdery mildew and black spot on roses. We tested a baking soda mix, chlorothalonil (a commercial fungicide), compost tea, horsetail soup, hydrogen peroxide, a mouthwash mix, a silicon injection treatment, a vinegar mix, a water treatment (we sprayed water on the plants once a week), and a control where nothing was applied. The results for each of these concoctions will be covered in their own entry. This test included two experiments, one on the rose cultivar *Rosa* 'Champlain', which is very susceptible to powdery mildew, and one on the rose cultivar *Rosa* 'Morden Centennial Pink', which is very susceptible to black spot. We performed this experiment under conditions of heavy pressure—in other words, we made sure that the plants were all exposed to black spot and powdery mildew.

Nine roses were tested for each concoction and cultivar. We looked at the plants 3 weeks after they were exposed to disease and rated them anywhere from a zero (no disease) to a five (completely covered with disease). At first glance, many of the home-brewed remedies that we tried were effective against powdery mildew, which certainly supports recommendations made by garden gurus. But while controlling powdery mildew is an admirable feat, you need to know one thing about the biology of powdery mildew before you get too excited. Powdery mildew hates water. It thrives in hot, dry conditions. If you went out twice a day, every day, and sprayed your roses off with water you would have very little powdery mildew; unfortunately, you might also encourage the onset of other diseases such as black spot.

While many of the homemade sprays we used did control powdery mildew to some extent, few performed better than a weekly spray of plain old water. Because of this it is safe to conclude that controlling powdery mildew is not the best test of a homemade fungicide's mettle. Rather, a better measure of how effectively these remedies control disease is to look at how well they control black spot.

Baking soda 🌱

Concoctions containing baking soda are advertised as being effective on a wide variety of diseases, the most common being powdery mildew. The use of baking soda is not new; the first published report of using baking soda to control diseases appeared in 1924 when Jesse Currey, a rose enthusiast, described his positive experience with it based on a recommendation made by the Russian plant pathologist Arthur de Yacxenski.

The practice

Most common baking soda recipes include about 1 tablespoon of baking soda per gallon of water, but some recipes include as much as 2 tablespoons per gallon of water. Additionally, most baking soda recipes include some quantity of soap and oil, usually 1 or 2 teaspoons of both per gallon of water.

The theory

Baking soda is supposed to disrupt fungal spores that land on the leaf surface, making them unable to infect the plant.

The real story

Baking soda has been used to control powdery mildew in a wide variety of plants, including euonymus, strawberry, cucurbits, and others (Ziv and Hagiladi 1993; Nam et al. 2003; Ziv and Zitter 1992). There is not much research on baking soda's ability to control diseases besides powdery mildew, but these sprays might affect diseases such as rust, dollar spot, and pythium blight (Moore 1996).

When we used baking soda to control black spot and powdery mildew on roses, we tested 1 tablespoon of baking soda in 1 gallon of water with about 1 teaspoon of dish soap added. We applied this concoction to our roses once per week. The mixture did not do much to control black spot, nor did it perform any better than water sprays in controlling powdery mildew. Why did we have such marginal results with powdery mildew when others have reported such good ones?

In 1992 a study tested baking soda alone and in combination with oil on powdery mildew in cucurbits (Ziv and Zitter). The study showed that baking soda alone, without the addition of oil, was ineffective at controlling this disease. Once oil was added, however, the mixture became very effective. Besides needing oil to make it effective, baking soda also needs to be applied at an early stage of infection, or even before you see any infection, to get the best results (Nam et al. 2003). In terms of baking soda's ability to control black spot, L. M. Massey reported in 1925 that it would probably not control this disease, so its failure in our tests was expected.

What it means to you ❀❀❀

Although our studies showed that baking soda was not more effective against powdery mildew than a once-a-week water spray, this is probably because we didn't add any type of oil with it. A tablespoonful of baking soda combined with 1 or 2 teaspoons of soap and 1 or 2 teaspoons of an oil, such as canola oil, mixed in a gallon of water is likely to help control disease on your plants; however, once you start adding soaps and oils to the baking soda you are greatly increasing the chance that you will damage your plants. Baking soda has the potential to burn plants all by itself, so be sure to test this concoction on similar plants before you treat anything of value.

Compost tea

Compost tea is an interesting idea that is finding some serious support from organic growers across the country. What's that? You've never heard of it? Okay, here's the lowdown. Compost tea is basically brewed by using a bucket as a kettle, a burlap sack (or something similar) as a teabag, and compost as the tea. Believe it or not this tea is usually served with sugar. The final product created by compost tea is supposed to be a soup of nutrients and, more importantly, beneficial bacteria that will help to defend your plants against disease.

The practice

The most basic compost teas are nothing but compost mixed with water and then filtered out to remove the solid portions. More complex, and supposedly better, ways to make compost tea can be purchased in kits. These kits include a sugar source (hopefully you remember how much bacteria and other microorganisms love sugar), a pail, an aeration device not unlike the air pump for a fishtank, and a "teabag," so that your compost can be suspended in water.

To get the kit working, you fill the pail with water and some of the sugar solution, add some compost to the teabag and suspend it in the water, and install the aerator in the pail to add oxygen to the mix—and off you go. This setup is supposed to allow bacteria, naturally growing in the compost, to move through the teabag and into the sugar water where they will feed, grow, and prosper. After a few days of letting the bacteria multiply in the bucket, the teabag is removed, and the water in the pail is ready to apply. Voilà! Compost tea.

Regardless of how compost teas are brewed they are usually applied by spraying them onto plants' foliage.

The theory

Two things are needed for compost tea to work as advertised. First, the bacteria present in compost must benefit plants by inhibiting pathogenic or "bad" fungi. Second, we must be able to culture these bacteria in the system that we are using.

The real story

Because compost tea is basically compost soaked in water, there is little doubt that some nutrients in the compost make it into the water. In terms of disease control, laboratory and greenhouse studies show compost tea to be somewhat effective at controlling bacterial spot on tomatoes and apple scab on petri dishes (Al-Dahmani et al. 2003; Cronin et al. 1996), but these results are not particularly dramatic and don't represent the type of application that would be made in the typical garden. More-typical tests of compost tea against diseases such as bacterial blight in carrots and late blight in tomatoes have shown this product to be ineffective (du Toit and Derie 2005; Inglis et al. 2004). In fact, by paging through *Fungicide and Nematicide Tests*, a journal devoted to pesticides and their effectiveness, you will quickly ascertain that compost tea seems to have little effect on any disease except powdery mildew, which sometimes seems to be controlled and sometimes seems to be made worse (McGrath 2004).

When we tested compost tea against black spot and powdery mildew on roses we found very little to indicate that it was particularly helpful in controlling these diseases. We used a commercially available kit, and we used compost composed mostly of old vegetative matter (weeds), which had been composting for about 6 months. We applied this tea to our roses as recommended—once a week for 2 weeks and then monthly.

Those who recommend compost tea typically point to its ability to control powdery mildew as evidence that this concoction is highly effective against disease. Before you start to believe these people be sure to reread the introduction to this section, being sure to take note of the fact that simply spraying water on plants can help ward off powdery mildew. In fact, spraying water on plants resulted in about the same level of powdery mildew control as our compost tea sprays. Black spot infection was not controlled by compost tea treatments at all.

Although the questionable results are certainly a reason not to use compost tea, I have a different concern: the presence of the beneficial microorganisms that it is supposed to supply. There is no doubt that microorganisms are present in these concoctions, but whether they will actually benefit plant growth and disease control depends upon the exact microorganisms that are in the tea, which is in turn dependent on how the tea was brewed, what materials were used for the brew, the microorganisms that you already have in your soil and on your plant, and what type of soil and plant you have in the first place. It is also entirely possible that human pathogens could live in the compost tea, depending on how it is brewed.

Compost teas can be made in a number of ways, and if you have your heart set on trying one, I recommend looking at the information presented by Dr. Elaine Ingham in her book *The Compost Tea Brewing Manual* (2000). Dr. Ingham is widely considered the world's expert on brewing compost teas. It is always to your benefit to use the best information possible when trying something that might or might not work, rather than just buying a compost tea kit and hoping for the best.

What it means to you ❀❀

Because of the many ways that compost teas are brewed and the lack of extensive research on each of those ways, it is difficult to tell exactly what compost tea will do for you or which type of compost tea to recommend. The research out there now seems to show nothing other than that the jury is still out on exactly what benefits can be expected from the various types of compost tea. I believe that compost tea has potential as both a source of nutrition and, perhaps, as a control for disease, so I won't say that it is a useless practice, but until more research is available I would avoid it.

Hydrogen peroxide

When you skin your elbow what is the first thing you look for? Hydrogen peroxide. Why? Because it kills microorganisms, thereby preventing your cut from getting infected. Can hydrogen peroxide protect your plants from disease as well?

The practice

Three percent hydrogen peroxide sprayed directly onto plants without dilution, or diluted to 50 percent, is recommended for controlling foliar diseases on a number of plants. Hydrogen peroxide is also sometimes recommended as an ingredient in some concoctions used to clean the roots of plants prior to planting. The most common recommendation for hydrogen peroxide is to spray this chemical undiluted once a week onto plants that you want to protect from disease.

The theory

Since hydrogen peroxide kills germs that infect humans it seems reasonable to assume that hydrogen peroxide can kill the germs that infect plants.

The real story

There is little doubt that hydrogen peroxide kills germs. This chemical has been used to kill microorganisms in a variety of different applications from sanitizing wounds to sanitizing fish eggs (Fitzpatrick et al. 1995). And yes, hydrogen peroxide has also been used to kill microorganisms on plants. In a study examining post-harvest grey mold in strawberries, hydrogen peroxide was applied to strawberries while they were growing in the field, and it did indeed affect the ability of grey mold to grow (Byun and Choi 2003). This was a post harvest experiment, however, meaning that the researchers were concerned with keeping strawberries disease free for a short time during and after harvest rather than for the life of the plant.

In our experiment with roses, we really didn't find too much to get excited about. We used a 3 percent hydrogen peroxide solution that we bought from the store and applied it at full strength once per week. This treatment was not particularly helpful for controlling either black spot or powdery mildew. Hopefully, you are asking yourself why the hydrogen peroxide wasn't helpful since we know that it kills microorganisms. The answer is actually pretty straightforward. Hydrogen peroxide is a relatively unstable chemical. Its chemical formula is H_2O_2. If that looks familiar to you, it's because it is very similar to the chemical formula for water: H_2O. Hydrogen peroxide breaks down quickly into water and oxygen and is unlikely to last on a plant for longer than a few hours even under the best conditions. A microorganism that takes up residence on a plant leaf soon after the hydrogen peroxide breaks down will have a week to become a full blown infection before the next application of hydrogen peroxide.

What it means to you ✿

Hydrogen peroxide is useful if all you want to do is sterilize something quickly, but it does not last long enough to give ongoing disease control in an outdoor environment.

Mouthwash

Mouthwash kills germs in your mouth using a wide variety of killing agents, including alcohol. Most recommendations that garden gurus make involving mouthwash are for killing diseases, and sometimes insects, on your plants.

The practice

Mouthwash is usually added to other things, such as tobacco or dish soap, to make a more complete spray. One commonly mentioned mixture suggests 1 part alcohol-containing mouthwash to 3 parts water. This mixture is then sprayed on your plants weekly as a disease control.

The theory

Since mouthwash is able to destroy microbes in your mouth it should do the same thing to microbes on plants.

The real story

Applying mouthwash to plants is not a particularly common recommendation among garden gurus, but it is out there. Mouthwash certainly has the potential to be effective as a fungicide simply because it is formulated to kill microbes. My biggest concern when applying it was the potential damage it could do to plants because of its relatively high concentration of alcohol.

The mouthwash mix we used included 1 cup of an ethanol-containing generic mouthwash along with 3 cups of water. We applied this concoction once per week to our plants. After a few weeks of observation, some very interesting results were observed. Mouthwash was head and shoulders better than the other homemade fungicides at controlling both powdery mildew and black spot. While it certainly wasn't as good as the commercial fungicide, it did do a much better job than I expected. The one drawback that we saw with mouthwash was that, when we first began to spray it on the young roses, it did cause the leaves to curl a little bit, but not nearly as badly as I thought it would.

What it means to you ❀❀❀

Mouthwash can actually work to help you fight disease on your plants, but there is a good chance it will cause some damage, too. If you really want to use mouthwash rather than a fungicide, which was actually created to control plant disease, then you had better be prepared to test whatever mouthwash you want to use on a plant you don't care much about before you start applying it to your prize-winning marigolds.

Those who tout mouthwash as an organic compound should think again. With ingredients such as cetylpyridinium chloride, domiphen bromide, and sodium saccharin, this homemade fungicide is something I would hesitate to call organic. That said, I was amazed at how well it performed in our test.

Silicon and horsetail soup

Silicon makes up over 25 percent of the earth's crust and is the primary ingredient in both sand and glass. Although silicon can be absorbed by many different types of plants, it is not considered an element that is required for plant life. Some plants are actually made up of as much as 10 percent silicon or more once you discount water (Ma et al. 2001). Recent research has shown that when plants are fertilized with silicon their ability to fight off disease can be enhanced. But do silicon protectants make sense for your garden? And can homemade silicon treatments such as horsetail soups, which use plants that contain high levels of silicon, be used instead?

The practice

Silicon protectants are applied either by spraying them onto foliage or by adding them to the soil. Instructions on the container usually result in an application of 100–150 parts per million of silicon in the irrigation water.

Horsetail (*Equisetum* spp.), a weed that accumulates silicon perhaps more efficiently than any other, can be made into a spray that is supposed to deliver silicon to plants. This spray is made by drying about ⅛–¼ cup of horsetails, crushing the dried leaves, boiling them in water, and then letting this soup simmer for 30 minutes. After simmering, the horsetail soup is ready to apply. Applications are usually made once a week to defend the plant from fungi.

The theory

There are currently two theories why silicon might protect plants from disease. The first, and most straightforward, is that silicon, being the primary component of glass, moves through a plant's vascular system to the leaves of the plant where it is deposited, thereby creating a glasslike barrier around the leaf. This glasslike barrier should help to repel diseases, and perhaps even insects, that try to infest the leaf. The second theory is that plants respond to additions of silicon by making phytoalexins. What are phytoalexins? They are the compounds that help plants fight off disease, kind of like our immune system.

The real story

It's interesting that we should have to add to our gardens an element that makes up 25 percent of the earth's crust. Why can't the plants get the stuff themselves? Actually there is an easy answer to that. Silicon is naturally present in the form of rocks and sand and, as anyone who has ever seen a beach can tell you, rocks and sand do not dissolve in water under normal conditions, except in extremely minute quantities. Protectants that include silicon in them get the silicon to dissolve in water by adding either sodium hydroxide or potassium hydroxide to powdered silicon dioxide (this is basically nothing more than crushed glass). The silicon dioxide will dissolve in the highly alkaline solution, and after it does water can be added to make a solution. The result is a liquid that contains silicon and, if potassium hydroxide was used, some potassium, too.

There has actually been quite a bit of research on the effects of silicon on a plant's ability to fight disease. Silicon has been effective for controlling disease in a number of crops, including grapes, cucumbers, and roses (Bowen et al. 1992; Cherif et al. 1994; Gillman et al. 2003). The biggest problem with using silicon as a disease control is that it must be applied daily and seems to have little or no effect if it is applied weekly. In our experiments on roses infected with black spot or powdery mildew, we found that silicon, applied daily along with irrigation water, was somewhat helpful for black spot but not so great for powdery mildew—and horsetail soup was basically good for nothing. The fact that the horsetail soup was not particularly helpful wasn't a great surprise. The silicon in the horsetails shouldn't be soluble in boiling water without the addition of potassium hydroxide or sodium hydroxide. If you broke a piece of glass into shards and boiled that in water you ought to have a spray about as effective as the horsetail soup. It is worth noting that some people find horsetails to be an effective scouring pad. Horsetails can be used in this way precisely because silicon doesn't dissolve in water.

The silicon injection's ability to help control black spot to some extent was not surprising considering some research we have conducted over the past few years (Gillman and Zlesak 2000), but I was disappointed that it didn't do better at controlling powdery mildew.

What it means to you ❀❀❀

Silicon injections and sprays are actually used by some botanic gardens, greenhouses, and nurseries to help them control disease, but these commercial growers and botanic gardens have the ability to apply silicon with most waterings, something that is not always easy for the typical gardener. Additionally, these outfits usually start using silicon before they ever see a problem and continue using the silicon for the entire growing season, something else that is not easy for the typical gardener. If you are willing to use silicon fertilizers before you see a problem and to add them with most of your waterings, silicon has some potential to help defend your plants against disease. If not, silicon probably isn't for you. Horsetail soup does not seem to be a reasonable alternative to using a commercial formulation of silicon and is barely worth a single flowerhead.

Vinegar as a fungicide

Vinegar was first noted as a fungicide in 1629 when it was recommended by John Parkinson, along with "cowes pisse, or cowes dung and urine," as a useful cure for tree canker. Vinegar was also once thought of as an effective insecticide. In 1833 William Kenrick presented hot vinegar as a remedy for aphids and certain other insect pests, something it is not well known for today. Vinegar is still an ingredient in some home-brewed disease controls, but it is less popular than many of the other ingredients, perhaps because it can burn plants if misapplied.

The practice

Apple cider vinegar is the most commonly applied vinegar for plant disease. About 2–3 tablespoons of this vinegar (usually containing 5 percent acetic acid) is mixed with 1 gallon of water to help control black spot and other diseases. Researchers working with vinegar have tried considerably higher concentrations.

The theory

Vinegar is a general poison that is damaging to plants and probably disease, too, courtesy of its high content of acetic acid.

The real story

Italian researchers examined vinegar as a fungicide in greenhouses to control powdery mildew on roses. Wine vinegar with a 6 percent acetic acid content was used in the experiment and applied in a 5 or 10 percent solution. This is considerably more than is usually recommended by the garden gurus. Three tablespoons of vinegar in a gallon of water is only about a 1 percent vinegar solution. In this same experiment acetic acid, the active antifungal chemical in vinegar, was also tested. Both the acetic acid and the vinegar, at all concentrations, were successful at controlling powdery mildew, but some plant damage was caused by the acetic acid (Pasini et al. 1997). Though wine vinegar was used in this test, there is no reason to believe that other vinegars, all of which contain acetic acid, shouldn't help to control powdery mildew.

Instead of wine vinegar we tested apple cider vinegar (a more common recommendation than wine vinegar, at least in the United States) against powdery mildew and black spot. This vinegar had 5 percent acidity, as is the case with many of the vinegars you buy off the grocery store shelf. We used 3 tablespoons of apple cider vinegar per gallon of water and applied the mixture to roses weekly. The vinegar turned out to be one of our weaker fungicides in terms of its ability to control black spot, but it proved to be just about equal to mouthwash in controlling powdery mildew. So basically, while our research agrees with other research on vinegar's ability to control powdery mildew, we are less impressed with its ability to control black spot. It is possible that if we had used higher concentrations of vinegar, or wine vinegar, as used by the Italian researchers, we would have had better luck.

What it means to you ❀❀

Vinegar fungicides may be effective on powdery mildew, but their ability to control other diseases is questionable to say the least. Since water sprays affect powdery mildew, too, I think I'd stick with something that affects more than just this easy-to-control disease. If you do decide to try vinegar, be aware that this spray has the potential to damage plants if too much is added to the mix, but also be aware that the more vinegar you add to the mix, the more likely you are to control powdery mildew and other diseases. If I were to try vinegar as a fungicide I would choose a plant that I was willing to sacrifice and try a variety of different vinegar concentrations on different portions of that plant to find out which varieties and concentrations were most effective at controlling disease without damaging the plant.

Putting it all together

The best way to control disease problems is to select plants that are resistant to diseases, to water your plants properly, and to fertilize them appropriately. If you do all these things then you have created conditions where few diseases should arise. When they do, however, it is best to be prepared with a plan for control.

Commercial choices

In our tests we never found anything superior to the commercial fungicide chlorothalonil. This fungicide has been around for a long time and is effective on a wide variety of diseases; additionally, not much resistance to this pesticide has been seen by researchers. Chlorothalonil's biggest drawback is that it coats plants with a whitish covering that many people find unattractive. There is a saying among golf course superintendents, "spray it white sleep at night," that provides an indication of how effective chlorothalonil is and of the color it gives to grass immediately after application. There are other commercial alternatives to this fungicide, but if I were to pick one out I would choose the organic fungicide neem. Other organic options include sulfur and Bordeaux mix, both of which are quite effective if used properly. Bordeaux mix can be toxic before it is mixed, so I steer away from it when possible. When working with commercial fungicides and other disease controls be sure to read the label very carefully and follow the recommended application methods.

Homemade choices

Our tests showed a few homebrews that, while not quite as effective as commercial fungicides, are certainly worth looking at. Mouthwash, though it caused some damage to plants, was almost as effective at controlling black spot and powdery mildew as chlorothalonil was. If I had to pick a home-brewed fungicide I would certainly consider using this one, while taking care not to apply too much and burn my plants. The other home-brewed remedy I would strongly consider is baking soda. While our tests didn't show that this home-brewed fungicide was particularly effective, adding a little bit of oil and soap has worked for other researchers. Do not expect baking soda to control black spot; it has been known for a long time that it won't. And be as careful with any homemade cure as you would with a commercial pesticide. Regardless of what they're made of, these remedies should not be considered completely safe for you or for your plants.

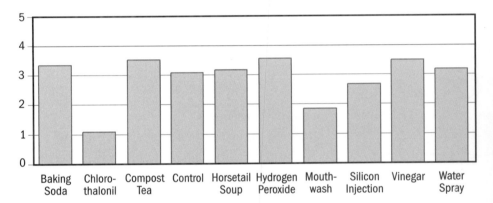

Figure 7. The prevalence of black spot on roses, from zero (no disease evident) to five (complete infestation). Nine treatments are compared to a control.

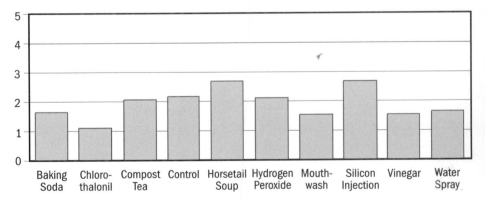

Figure 8. The prevalence of powdery mildew on roses, from zero (no disease evident) to five (complete infestation). Nine treatments are compared to a control.

7

Herbicides

SINCE PREHISTORIC times people have tried to prevent plants from growing where they don't want them—with varying degrees of success. There is no doubt that commercial pesticides offer the surest way to kill plants, but there are also many practices promoted by garden gurus, and even university personnel, that might work for your garden, depending on exactly what you are looking for. Most of the herbicides in this section are broad spectrum poisons, meaning they kill plants indiscriminately. If you want to conserve certain plants, such as grass, and kill others, such as dandelions, then you will probably need to resort to some of the products in chapter 9.

Brussels sprouts for bad plants

Some plants, such as black walnut, contain chemicals that inhibit other plants from growing nearby. Some people believe that grinding up plants that have these chemicals in them and placing them on soil can help to keep that soil free from weeds. Furthermore, they say that this can be done with much less material than you would need for typical mulch. The list of plants that they claim work best for this includes Brussels sprouts, broccoli, cabbage, canola, and other plants in the genus *Brassica*.

The practice

The standard recommendation for using *Brassica* as an herbicide includes mixing these plants in a blender with some water and applying the slurry to areas where you want to control weeds.

The theory

Plants in the genus *Brassica* are supposed to contain chemicals that inhibit the growth of seedlings, so if they are applied before weed seeds sprout, they should be able to prevent the growth of these weeds.

The real story

There are a number of reasons to believe that ground Brussels sprouts and other related plants will work to control weeds. The first reason is personal experience. If you have ever planted a field of canola (OK, I realize that not too many of you have done this) you will know that weeds just don't seem to like to grow around this plant. That's good news for the gardener, because it means that maybe, just maybe, there is something in canola and its close relatives that could help to control weeds.

Extracts from broccoli have been shown to inhibit the germination of seeds (Brown and Morra 1995) and the growth of roots (deFeo et al. 1997). Other plants in the genus *Brassica* have also been reported to help control soil-borne microorganisms that might affect crops. Most plants in this genus have a group of chemical compounds called glucosinolates, which is the apparent reason behind this ability. Though glucosinolates are not particularly effective at controlling weeds themselves, they break down into other chemicals called isothiocyanates, which are poisonous to a wide variety of things, including microbes and plants (Rosa and Rodrigues 1999), and could potentially be used as a way to control weeds. (Notice the suffix on that last chemical: cyanate—think cyanide.)

There is little doubt that, because of isothiocyanates, plants in the genus *Brassica* may be beneficial for weed control. However, this weed control may not be quite as perfect as we would hope. If you incorporate these plants into the ground with a tiller, hoping to get long-term weed control, you will probably be disappointed. In one experiment, tilling one type of *Brassica* (rapeseed) into the soil didn't stop peas from germinating when it was tilled in just 19 days before the peas were planted (Al-Khatib et al. 1997). Other research is even more discouraging. In one laboratory study a group of researchers found that 90 percent of isothiocyanates break down within 48 hours of being applied to soil. This breakdown is at least somewhat weather dependant, with wetter, warmer conditions resulting in more rapid breakdown. These researchers also found that smaller seeds are more likely to be affected by isothiocyanates than larger seeds (Peterson et al. 2001).

I tested ground canola (*Brassica napus*) to see if it would inhibit the growth of seeds. In my experiment I filled two trays with potting media; planted corn, beans, and radishes in each; and applied a slurry of freshly ground canola and a very small amount of water (enough to moisten the leaves before grinding) to one of the trays. What I found was rather disappointing. There was no difference at all between the germination of seeds in either of the trays, and the plants in the trays with the canola slurry actually ended up growing better, probably because of the added nutrition that the ground canola offered. When I have planted canola in the field I have been impressed by how well it discourages weeds. Obviously, when this plant is harvested and ground up, its effectiveness as a weed control is greatly diminished.

What it means to you ❀❀

Using plants in the genus *Brassica* to control weeds might work for a short time if they are tilled into the ground, but grinding up these plants and using the slurry to control weeds doesn't seem to hold much promise. Even plants that are grown and then tilled into the soil don't offer long term weed control. A good commercial herbicide that might be appropriate if you need this type of control is trifluralin.

Corn gluten meal

A preemergent herbicide is one that affects the growth of a plant before it emerges from the soil, thereby stopping the problem before it starts. Once the plant emerges from the soil preemergent herbicides will rarely have any effect on it. Preemergent herbicides have, until recently, been composed primarily of synthetic compounds. In January 1990 Dr. Nick Christians of Iowa State University filed for a patent. The title of this patent was *Preemergence Weed Control Using Corn Gluten Meal*, and in 1991 we had a natural preemergent weed control.

The practice

Corn gluten meal is sold at many garden centers and is usually applied to the surface of the soil at a concentration of 12 to 20 pounds per 1000 square feet.

The theory

Corn gluten meal is supposed to contain chemicals that inhibit the germination of seeds from other plants. It is also supposed to be safe for plants that have already emerged from the soil. Corn gluten meal, because it is a formerly living thing, lends some fertility to the area where it is applied and is commonly advertised as containing about 10 percent nitrogen.

The real story

The reason that corn gluten meal works as a preemergent herbicide is that it contains a group of chemicals, the most important of which is probably alaninyl-alanine, that inhibit young root growth (Unruh et al. 1997).

Most research on corn gluten meal has been accomplished in the upper Midwest. This research shows that it is effective against a wide variety of weeds such as nightshade, lambsquarter, bentgrass, and a host of others (Bingaman and Christians 1995). Research in California produced results that were somewhat different, though, with corn gluten meal having little effect on weeds (Wilen et al. 1999). It is possible that the different climates in these locations affect corn gluten meal's effectiveness. It is also possible that different types of soils or media could affect the ability of corn gluten meal to work effectively.

Although extensive research has not been published, I have had the opportunity to talk with some landscapers about this product, and they claim that corn gluten meal is an effective preemergent herbicide if you are willing to apply it to the same site for at least 2 or 3 years and to put up with weeds during that time. These landscapers also claim that corn gluten meal is an excellent fertilizer and may help to control weeds in a lawn simply by invigorating the grass, which then crowds the weeds right out. Indeed, if corn gluten meal is applied at a rate of 20 pounds per 1000 square feet it should supply enough nitrogen to so that other fertilizers will not be necessary.

What it means to you ✤✤✤

If all you want to do is to control weeds before they emerge, some fantastic synthetic preemergent herbicides will accomplish what you want. If, on the other hand, you want to control weeds before they emerge, but you want to use a natural method, you are left with one of three things: mulch, corn gluten meal, or Brussels sprouts. Mulch will give you faster control but will break down; corn gluten meal will work, but you have to wait a few years; Brussels sprouts don't seem to work well and certainly won't last long.

Mulch the magnificent 🐾

Mulching around a tree to prevent weed growth and to increase the moisture of the soil is an old practice. Nineteenth-century gardeners indicated that they could increase production anywhere from 15 to 25 percent simply by mulching (William 1871b). Back in the days before herbicides, mulches were the best control available for weeds, but how do they fare today?

The practice

Mulches can be made of almost anything, but the most common mulches include wood chips, gravel, and plastic. The basic guidelines for mulching plants involve spreading the mulch around the tree or shrub to a depth of about 2–3 inches. It is usually recommended that the mulch be at least 3–4 inches from the stem of the tree or shrub, so the resulting shape is that of a donut.

The theory

Mulch supposedly creates an almost impenetrable barrier to young plants wherever it is placed, thereby excluding weeds from the area where your plant's roots will grow to pick up nutrients and moisture. Besides excluding weeds, mulch is also supposed to provide a barrier to evaporation, allowing the soil to retain its moisture more effectively.

The real story

Mulch is very effective at what it is supposed to do. There are many types of mulch, though, and they all have strengths and weaknesses. Inorganic mulches, such as rocks, tend to be less effective at weed control, depending on how deep the mulched layer is, but they do aid in keeping soils moist for a longer period of time (Walker and Powell 2001). In terms of weed control the best, easy-to-get mulch is probably straw. Straw is superior to other mulches not only because it inhibits weed growth but also because it attracts birds, whose activity can disturb the soil where the weeds are trying to establish themselves (Hartley and Rahman 1997). Sawdust is also a good mulch and is equal to straw in many ways, but it likely will not control some grasses as effectively (Hartley and Rahman 1997). Yard wastes are some of the most common mulches used and, indeed, can be very effective. However, studies that looked at yard waste with a large proportion of grass clippings have shown that, if you are applying herbicides to your grass to control weeds, the mulch that you make from these treated grass clippings can have negative effects on the growth of the plants that you mulch (Bahe and Peacock 1995). But herbicides are not the only problem with yard clippings. Grasses actually contain some chemicals that inhibit the growth of other plants. While those chemicals are certainly useful when you're trying to control weeds, they're not nearly as attractive when you're wondering why your tomato seeds didn't sprout (Buta et al. 1987). Grass is not the best mulch for newly planted or seeded areas. Let your plants get established before using it.

Synthetic mulches, including polyethylene sheets that create barriers to weed growth, are becoming more popular. Using polyethylene sheets alone, or even under rock mulch, will provide very effective weed control; however, polyethylene will probably not be as effective as straw mulches at helping to retain soil moisture (Hedau and Kumar 2002). Polyethylene mulches actually block water from reaching the ground, unlike organic mulches, which allow water to percolate through and eventually reach the soil below. Although cutting holes in the polyethylene can offer a solution, weeds tend to grow through the holes the first chance they get.

The biggest problem with organic mulches is that they will decompose over time. After a few years, your mulch actually ends up as compost. This happens most quickly with mulches that are finely ground or rich in nutrients. Mulches such as farmyard litter and grass clippings tend to break down very rapidly. Though farmyard litter inhibits weeds and helps the soil to retain moisture better than many other mulches (Uniyal and Mishra 2003), it is probably not the best choice for most situations.

What it means to you ✿✿✿✿✿

Mulch is very useful and accomplishes exactly what it is supposed to. Choosing a mulch that fits your needs is important. Rock mulches will not control weeds as well as most other mulches, but they will last for a long time. Organic mulches are very effective at controlling weeds and at allowing water to reach the plants, but they will eventually break down. Polyethylene mulches are very effective at blocking weeds, but can block water from reaching the ground and are not very attractive without something else, usually gravel, placed on top.

Salt ☿

Perhaps the oldest known herbicide is salt or, more specifically, salt and ashes. This concoction was used in Roman times to sterilize the fields of the enemies of Rome at the end of the Third Punic War. (Actually, historians dispute whether this was actually done; nonetheless, the mention of using salt as an herbicide in old documents indicates that for quite some time, salt has been known to destroy plant life.) Somewhat later, in the early 1900s, salt was recommended as a way to control weeds in asparagus, a crop that is notoriously resistant to salt poisoning (Walker 1905). In the U.K., salt has been labeled for use as an herbicide in sugar beets (United Kingdom 1985). It has also been considered as a way to help control some diseases (Russel 1978), though using sodium chloride in this way is currently quite rare. Most modern recommendations for weed control do not include this herbicide, and even garden gurus tend to avoid it.

The practice

Salt, also known as sodium chloride, is applied to the soil at a high concentration to kill weeds. Salt is usually used as a solid, without dissolving it in water, though there are some commercial organic herbicides that mix sodium chloride, vinegar, and water to make a spray-on herbicide. A cup of salt per 10 square feet should kill plants nicely, but more could be added if this does not yield satisfactory results.

The theory

Salt draws water out of plant cells and, by doing so, should cause the plant to desiccate and eventually die.

The real story

The activity of sodium chloride on plants is very straightforward. When a solution of salt outside the plant's cells is more concentrated than the solution of salt inside the plant's cells, the plant will lose water through osmosis, desiccate, and die. This can even happen when the plant grows in a large amount of water. Every year I demonstrate to one of my classes how salt can kill a plant. I grow plants hydroponically and add various amounts of sodium chloride to the hydroponic solutions. It is very interesting to watch. With no sodium chloride added the plant will be perfectly healthy, with a small amount of sodium chloride there will be some wilting, and with a large amount death will occur. Besides the desiccation salt causes, the elements sodium and chlorine are both toxic to plants at high-enough levels.

Salt is a contact herbicide, so it will not travel in a plant's vascular system and will only affect the part of the plant that it touches. If salt is used as a spray, it is likely to kill the shoots of the plant and leave the roots alive, resulting in the weed's resprouting from the roots.

What it means to you ❀❀

If even the garden gurus don't recommend it, that ought to give you a hint as to how potentially bad this stuff is for your garden. If you just want to knock out a weed or two, salt is probably fine, but placing a large amount of salt on your ground is not a good idea because it may hurt other nearby plants or plants that you plan on placing there in the future.

Vinegar as an herbicide

Vinegar is listed in this book three times, once as a soil acidifier, once as a fungicide, and once as an herbicide or plant killer. If vinegar was an incredibly effective herbicide would it also be listed as a fungicide and a fertilizer? It all seems kind of fishy to me.

The practice
Vinegar is applied to weeds at a concentration of anywhere from 5 percent to 100 percent. The most commonly recommended vinegars include apple cider vinegar and white vinegar.

The theory
Vinegar is high in acetic acid, which is supposed to kill plants.

The real story
Vinegar is not a particularly well-researched herbicide. To get a little data on how effective it might be we sprayed undiluted vinegar, vinegar mixed with an equal amount of water, and a solution that was 80 percent water and 20 percent vinegar onto a few small plots that included grass, clover, dandelions, and some other weeds. We used white vinegar with an acid content of 5 percent. The first time we performed this experiment it rained about an hour after we applied the vinegar. In this situation only the 100 percent vinegar solution had much effect on the plants. When we repeated the experiment the next day using new plots, we found, unsurprisingly, that the vinegar was much more effective when it was allowed to sit on the weeds for a little longer before being washed off.

Plots treated with 100 percent vinegar were really knocked for a loop. Most plants in them turned brown within 2 days. Plants in the plots treated with 50 percent vinegar also had significant damage, but less than those treated with 100 percent vinegar and not enough to satisfy most people. Plants treated with 20 percent vinegar had some damage, but nothing that a few days couldn't cure. The most interesting result we observed was the tendency for plants that appeared to have been killed by vinegar to grow back within a week or two. The reason for this is that vinegar is a contact poison, meaning that it kills the parts of the plant that it touches but doesn't affect the parts that it doesn't touch. Because we applied the vinegar with a sprayer the roots were not touched, and they rapidly sent up new shoots. If vinegar is poured on the ground the roots can be killed, but it takes a lot of vinegar. Just applying a few drops to the ground will not do it.

What it means to you ❀❀❀

Household vinegar is an effective contact herbicide when it is applied directly to a plant without being diluted, but because it is a contact poison it will not kill plant roots unless it is applied extremely heavily. Some plants that may have appeared dead at first will regrow. Dousing the ground with a large amount of vinegar will kill plant roots, but it seems to be quite wasteful to me, especially when commercial herbicides, such as glyphosate, will do a better job with less.

Putting it all together

Some very effective methods are available for controlling weeds without using synthetic commercial herbicides, and some synthetic commercial herbicides work so well you wonder why you even tried anything else. It all comes down to how you want to control your weeds. Around my house I like to use the organic methods whenever I can, but at work sometimes these just aren't effective enough.

Controlling weeds before they pop up

Quite an assortment of things can be done to control weeds before they jump out of the ground and surprise you. I prefer organic methods whenever possible, and fortunately, there are some great ones out there. Bar none, mulch is the best weed control if you are in a situation where you can use it. Mulch has the advantage of offering not only weed control but also improved water availability, and as the mulch rots it will even offer compost. Mulch does not lend itself to all situations, though, primarily because of the need for transportation.

When mulch isn't an option, the grower who wants to use organics might consider corn gluten meal. Corn gluten meal is a relatively new product that is useful for controlling weeds when applied at a fairly heavy dose. It is not particularly effective in its first year, but given 2 or 3 years it may work well. Although other preemergent weed controls are tried periodically, no current homebrews can reliably control weeds before they emerge.

Many synthetic commercial herbicides can hinder the emergence of unwanted plants in your garden. The most common of these include trifluralin and siduron. Trifluralin affects many different types of weeds and can be expected to work for a number of months. Siduron will not last as long but is considered a good product because it does not usually affect the seeds of grasses used in temperate climates.

Controlling weeds after they sprout

The best way to control weeds after they sprout is certainly hand weeding. Most people don't like to hand weed large areas, though, so they look for other options. For the person looking to control their weeds organically there are a few reasonable choices. The first is a flamethrower. I do not consider these contraptions particularly safe, but there is little doubt that they work. You can purchase them from many farm supply shops, and they comprise nothing more than a hose running from a propane tank to a nozzle from which the flammable gas is released. Flames definitely inhibit the ability of the plants to grow but do not always affect the roots because soil makes an excellent insulator. If splashing flames around your garden doesn't sound like the way you'd like to spend a relaxing Saturday consider two other possible options. Salt will kill weeds, but it is also likely to make your soil less able to support desirable plants, as few of them like salty soils, asparagus being an exception. Vinegar is another option that is generally much safer. Vinegar will kill the parts of the weed that it comes into contact with, but it is unlikely to do much to the roots. The more concentrated the vinegar is, the more successful you will be at eliminating weeds. One hundred percent vinegar will be the most successful option, but you can probably achieve some control down to a 50 percent mix of vinegar and water if you are using vinegar with 5 percent acidity or greater.

If you decide that a homebrew isn't for you and you want to use a well-established commercial herbicide there are many to choose from. Two of the better postemergent herbicides that were created to kill just about any green plant include glyphosate and glufosinate-ammonium. Both of these herbicides will leave the area that you treat a nice, crispy brown. If you are looking for a commercial organic herbicide, those that include garlic oil (and sometimes vinegar) tend to be effective but do not always kill the roots. If, on the other hand, you are interested in killing broadleaf weeds (basically this means weeds that are not grasses), you might consider 2,4-D, or a combination of 2,4-D, mecoprop (MCPP), and dicamba. These mixes are extremely effective on broadleaf plants such as clover, dandelion, and plantain, but are not particularly harmful to most grasses. They are found in many weed and feed mixtures for grass and are often also sold as sprays. If you are looking to kill unwanted grass, such as crabgrass, a few herbicides might prove very effective, such as MSMA (monosodium acid methanearsonate) and calcium acid methanearsonate. These chemicals tend to be very effective in killing annual grasses, but safe for many (but not all) perennial grasses. Always be very careful when using selective herbicides, and read the label to make sure you are not targeting the very thing you want to save.

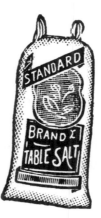

8

Other Pesticides and Protectants

A HUGE NUMBER of products and practices control things other than insects, diseases, and weeds. They include deer and rodent repellents, slug controls, and products to control problems related to environmental conditions, such as sun scald. As with the other products and practices we have looked at, some are founded on firm scientific footing and some are just ridiculous.

Bagging fruit

Putting a bag around fruits while they are still on a tree or vine seems like a lot of work, but people have started doing this for many different fruits, including apples, pears, and others. The practice actually started in Asia and found its way to the U.S. relatively recently. Bagging fruit is supposed to protect it from all kinds of nasty insects and diseases.

The practice

Some sort of a bag, usually plastic, is placed on the fruit of a tree soon after the fruit starts to mature (while it is $\frac{1}{2}$ inch or so in diameter). Some people actually purchase something called a Japanese apple bag. These bags are reported to work quite well and are specifically designed for placing onto fruit trees. The bag is stapled shut, or a twist tie is used to affix it firmly around the fruit. It is best to have the bag tightly sealed so excess water and small pests cannot get into it. Bags are usually left on the fruit until about 3 weeks before harvest to ensure that the fruit ripens properly and is not off-color.

The theory

Bags surrounding fruits are thought to provide a physical barrier to diseases and insects while the fruit matures.

The real story

Most published research on bagging fruit has been done in China and other Asian countries. Research has generally been on apples, but other fruits such as kiwis and grapes have also shown benefits from bagging (Jing 2003; Wang 2003; Xin and Zhang 2003). The research shows that bagging fruit is extremely beneficial to fruit quality, but no studies have shown a complete elimination of problems. Leaving the bag on throughout ripening will help to further protect the fruit, but the fruit will probably not develop its normal color and texture if the covering is not taken off about 2–3 weeks before the fruit is ready to be harvested.

Although there has not been nearly as much work done in the U.S. or Europe as there has in the Far East, some Westerners have tried this practice. In 2000 Larry Zilliox, a researcher in Minnesota, compared a few different types of bags, including paper bags, zip-lock bags, plastic film, and some others in their ability to protect apples. He covered the fruit after it was about the size of a quarter and kept the bags on over the course of the entire season. He found that the zip-lock bags made the most sense because they were easy to find and use and that it was best to staple them shut. He also found that water tends to collect in bags after rains; though this water didn't harm the fruit, the increased weight of the bag could damage the limb, so it makes sense to drain the water by cutting off the bottom corners of the bag (small cuts are probably best). This method produced fruit with excellent size and flavor.

What it means to you ❀❀❀❀❀

If you have the inclination to spend your time bagging fruit, you will be rewarded. It does work. Don't think it is a cure-all—problems can and do occur—but when this method is used, overall fruit quality is usually quite high.

Beer as a slug killer

Placing a saucer of beer beside your plants to protect them from slugs might be one of the most well-known homemade pest control measures ever devised. But is it really the best method for getting rid of slugs?

The practice

A saucer full of beer near plants you want to protect from slugs is a highly touted remedy. Most people recommend old stale beer, but some recommend a higher-end brew. A slightly more refined recommendation to catch these slimy pests includes digging a small hole and inserting a bowl or jar into it so that the lip of the bowl is even with the surface of the soil. Beer is then added up to an inch or so below the lip of the bowl.

The theory

Beer is supposed to attract slugs to the beer-filled container. They try to get into the container to ingest the beer, fall in, and drown. Drowning in beer—I had some old college friends—no, wait, this isn't that kind of book.

The real story

Beer traps are actually an accepted way to measure slug populations for scientific studies, the one problem being that slug traps are somewhat species specific: some types of slugs are attracted to beer more than other types (Voss et al. 1998). Additionally, a poorly designed beer trap will attract a slug without actually trapping it. This could be bad news for plants in the area. A poorly designed trap is one where the slug has a difficult time getting into the beer to drown itself. A prime example would be a bowl with sides that flare out and are slick. A slug would have a tough time climbing this barrier and might become enamored with a nearby patch of hostas instead. When I have placed beer traps on top of the ground I have been very disappointed.

What it means to you ✿✿✿✿

Beer traps are a useful and easy way to control slugs, just be careful to set up your traps so that the slugs are caught and not just attracted. The top of your trap should be even with the surface of the soil, and the level of beer in the container should be about an inch below the top of the trap so the slugs have to extend their bodies to reach it; as they extend they will fall in and drown. The best containers to use are those that are deep enough to allow an inch of clearance at the top while still having enough room for 5–6 inches of beer. If traps aren't set properly then you can expect slugs to come for the beer and stay for the very plants you're trying to protect.

Deer and rodent repellents from your blender

Repelling mammals isn't really that hard. Just find something that smells offensive to you, and it will be offensive to other creatures. Rotten eggs, garlic, rotten meat, onions, urine, and other things that you are happy to get out of your home have been offered as ways to keep deer and rodents out of your garden. They will certainly have that effect on friends, family, and neighbors, which may or may not be a good thing, depending on how long you like people to linger at your garden parties.

The practice

A number of surefire (the gurus' word, not mine) methods are suggested to repel deer and rodents from your garden. Some involve hanging soap, garlic, or something else distasteful near your plants; some involve planting only deer resistant trees and shrubs; and some involve mixing foul-smelling concoctions into a spray that can be applied to plants. Here is a slightly modified recipe taken from a 1998 issue of *Consumer Reports*. Mix four eggs, 2 ounces of red pepper sauce, and 2 ounces of chopped garlic in a 1-quart container, and then add enough water to fill. Blend this concoction, and strain out the solids. Apply the resulting liquid to plants to protect them from deer. Some people suggest adding antitranspirants to the spray to allow the repellent to stay on the plant for a longer period of time.

The theory

Smell and taste are very powerful senses. If these senses are assailed with nasty-smelling and -tasting treatments, deer and rodents might keep away from our plants.

The real story

Various stunt-based game shows on TV have utilized the extreme power of taste and smell in their stunts. Some of the more disgusting feats people have had to accomplish include ingesting repulsive food items, such as rotten eggs and cockroaches. Obviously no one wants to eat these things, but in the face of a great reward, most people do. Though the food tastes and smells disgusting, it's worth the pain to receive the prize. Rodents and deer faced with repellents act in much the same way. If a food item (in this case a tree or shrub) is coated with, or located near, something disgusting or distasteful, the animal will avoid it unless it's worth the reward. Over the winter months when little food is available, the reward that an animal receives for eating something distasteful is life. I don't think I'm stretching the truth when I say that most people would eat a rotten egg to avoid starving to death. Conclusion? No repellent is ever going to be perfect, and you shouldn't expect them to be.

Hanging bars of soap from your trees is an easy way to keep mammals, and especially deer, away from your yard without using sprays or particularly nasty-smelling concoctions. Experiments conducted by R. K. Swihart and M. R. Conover (1990) showed that an area extending about 1 meter (1.09 yards) from the soap will be protected from deer, though this protection is not perfect and some damage should still be expected. Their experiment further showed that, despite common wisdom, there is no bar soap that is significantly better than another for repelling deer.

The most common constituents of homemade mammal-repelling sprays are garlic, hot peppers, and rotten eggs. These items are similar to the ingredients present in many commercial repellents. In fact, in *Consumer Reports*'s tests (1998), the homemade spray was as repellent to deer as commercial sprays were. It also found that soap and hair hung from trees was reasonably effective, concluding that "using almost any repellent is better than using nothing." It should be noted, though, that in this experiment researchers encountered low overall deer pressure, making it difficult to definitively establish the efficacy of the various treatments.

Other natural repellents have been tested for protecting susceptible plants from deer and other grazing animals. These include hot pepper sauce, daffodil bulbs, catnip, *Iris* rhizomes, and peppermint (Ries et al. 2001). Extracts from all these plants and plant products were effective at repelling deer, rabbits, and squirrels to one degree or another; unfortunately, in this experiment extracts were mixed with various solvents that would not be healthy to most plants in a garden and that are not even available to most people because of the potential risks involved in using them.

Extracts generally proved to be effective for 2 weeks or less, with the exception of a catnip extract that lasted for 32 days, which is comparable to commercial deer repellents. It is easily conceivable that these different products could be mixed up or blended in a way that is safe and that would be effective in repelling deer at a much lower cost than a commercial deer repellent.

What it means to you ❀❀❀

There is no reason to think that a homemade deer repellent will be any less effective than a commercial repellent. They often use very similar ingredients, but it is important to remember that under extreme pressure deer and rodents will ignore any repellent. Deer and rodent repellents, both homemade and commercial, need to be reapplied frequently to maintain an acceptable level of repellency. Adding an antitranspirant to your homemade mix might help to keep the mix on your plants for a longer period of time, but it might also burn the plants' foliage or bark. If you want to mix antitranspirants with anything be sure to test the spray on an expendable plant first.

Deer and rodent repellents from the store

Repellents for various mammalian pests are some of the most widely used and demanded gardening products around the world, and creative inventors and entrepreneurs have been trying to make money off them for years. Take, for example, a formulation to repel rats patented in 1899 by Eben Dowie and James Oxley. This concoction included 20 percent chili powder, 5 percent hellebore, 8 percent sulphate of lime, 8 percent phosphate of lime, 54 percent carbonate of lime, and 5 percent oxide of iron. The inventors claimed that the first two ingredients were the active ones and made a note that a type of coal could substitute for the last four. It's interesting that modern producers of commercial repellents are still using chilies or other hot peppers as one of the major components of their formulations.

The practice

Most repellents are designed to be applied to bark or foliage, usually with a handheld sprayer. They contain a variety of ingredients, including but not limited to egg whites, garlic, castor oil, the urine of predatory animals, and capsaicin (hot pepper sauce).

The theory

Repellents are foul smelling or foul tasting natural products or, sometimes, synthetic chemicals. They are sprayed onto plants in the hopes that deer will avoid them.

The real story

Most commercial repellents are usually about as effective as homemade repellents, which makes a lot of sense because they usually have the same basic ingredients. Ideally, a commercial product offers a foul-tasting mix that does not wash off of your trees or shrubs as quickly as a home-brewed repellent would. This is accomplished with various oils and waxes (such as antitranspirants) that most consumers would not have easy access to. Indeed, in experiments where commercial repellents were evaluated for longevity, they typically lasted longer than homemade repellents would be expected to, maintaining their effectiveness for up to 12 weeks (Conover 1987; Swihart and Conover 1990).

Commercial repellents have different abilities to ward off deer and rodents, depending on the product used, location, and number of four-footed (or -hoofed) pests in the area. An experiment in Michigan investigated the commercial repellents Tree Guard, Bobbex, Hinder, and Miller's Hot Sauce in their ability to keep squirrels, deer, and rabbits away from ears of corn and white cedar branches. In this experiment no commercial formulation managed to repel animals for longer than a few days (Ries et al. 2001). In Rhode Island an evaluation of the commercial deer repellents Deer Away, Holly Ridge, Tree Guard, Bobbex, and Deer Off noted that these products performed well under low-feeding-intensity conditions but not as well under higher-intensity conditions, though Deer Away and Holly Ridge fared better than the rest. Both of these products include putrescent egg solids in their formulation (Lemieux et al. 2000). Even in this study, where commercial repellents were effective for 8–12 weeks (albeit with variable deer pressure), the authors note that it is possible they would not be able to prevent deer damage over an entire winter because the products require multiple applications at temperatures above 45 degrees Fahrenheit (7 degrees Celsius). In northern regions it is quite likely that an acceptable temperature would not occur at the scheduled reapplication time.

In a small experiment conducted in Minnesota during the winter of 1999 we applied a variety of commercial deer and rodent repellents to a small grouping of sand cherries. As you can imagine, there is quite a lack of food for little critters in Minnesota during the winter months. We treated these cherries one time at the beginning of winter (November) with the commercial repellents Tree Guard, Hinder, and Ro-pel and also left a few plants untreated. Our primary pests were voles, mice, and rabbits. Every month we went out to check how effective the repellents had been in keeping critters away from our plants, but at no time were any of the repellents more effective than the control. Unfortunately, people who do not reapply deer and rodent repellents find the same results. In missing a scheduled reapplication time or, in our case, not reapplying repellents at all (when it's −10 degrees Fahrenheit outside, it's difficult to spray), you might as well not have applied anything in the first place. Repellent products are likely to wear off after a few weeks because of wind, rain, snow, and other environmental factors.

What it means to you ❀❀❀

Commercial repellents for deer and rodents may work, but they are generally most effective under conditions of low feeding pressure and are rarely effective for more than a short period of time. Reapplications usually need to be made anywhere from 2 to 12 weeks after the initial application. Repellents containing putrescent egg solids (rotten eggs) seem to perform consistently better than others. Before considering an over-the-counter repellent, you would be wise to at least consider a homemade repellent because they are likely to be just as effective as commercial repellents, though reapplication might need to be more frequent.

Eggshells for slug fencing

Using crushed eggshells as a barrier to deter slugs from reaching a plant is a common recommendation. The eggshells are supposed to produce something like a barbed wire fence around the plants, thereby blocking the slugs from reaching them.

The practice

Eggshells are crushed and placed around valuable plants. Most recommendations do not mention how deep or how wide the eggshell fence should be but do imply that it should be as deep and wide as possible.

The theory

There is a commercial organic pesticide called diatomaceous earth that is composed of the skeletons of microscopic organisms called diatoms. These skeletons are made of silicon and are extremely sharp; in fact, they are literally shards of glass. Slugs prefer not to crawl over this pesticide, but if they do, they cut themselves, sometimes fatally. Because of the sharp edges on crushed eggshells, slugs might behave the same way around them that they would around diatomaceous earth.

The real story

Besides one paragraph write-ups in home remedy magazines and books, there really isn't much information out there regarding how well eggshells work as a slug fence. With this in mind I prepared a small trial to check it out.

I bought some paper plates and eggs from the grocery store, as well as some limes and whipped cream. My wife set about making lime pies, and I went about cleaning, drying, and crushing eggshells. After crushing the eggshells, I placed them in a ring around the edge of the plate and put some slugs in the center. This is an impossible test of course because I knew the slugs would eventually exit the plate. I planned to measure how long it would take slugs to exit the plate surrounded with eggshells as opposed to a plate without eggshells. In theory the slugs should take longer to exit a plate surrounded with eggshells because they are deterred by the shells' sharp edges. Unfortunately, I never needed to test a plate without eggshells because the slugs were so completely undeterred. Fearing that I hadn't crushed the eggshells enough, I reran this experiment with eggshells that were anywhere from slightly crushed to very crushed (using a rolling pin) and I also varied the depth of the pile of shells. At a moderately crushed level (pieces were about the size of a baby aspirin) applied to a depth of 1/4 inch or more, the eggshells slowed the slugs. That is not to say the slugs were reluctant, because they weren't, but they had a tougher time getting through the shells than when the pile was thin and the eggshell chunks were thick. When the eggshell pieces were at other sizes, the slugs had an easier time navigating their way across the barrier.

After running this experiment I was a bit surprised. I try not to have any major preconceived notions about the results of my experiments, but that wasn't the case with eggshells. I honestly expected them to work and was rather disappointed when they didn't. I immediately became afraid that the whole concept of putting something small and sharp around your plants to protect them might be a waste of time, so I purchased some diatomaceous earth, and tested it in the same way. I needn't have worried. The slugs quite clearly hated the stuff. One bolted off the plate in the first 10 minutes. (This was a sad and pitiful thing to watch because he was constantly winding and rolling, trying to get away from the sharp substance under his foot. If I had any sympathy for slugs I would have helped him, but I don't, so I didn't.) The other six slugs remained confined to the plate after 3 hours. When I again checked the plate after 12 hours all the slugs had left with the exception of one, which had perished. At this point I feel rather confident saying diatomaceous earth works as advertised.

What it means to you ❀❀

Eggshells crushed to the size of baby aspirin and applied relatively deeply around your plants could inhibit the movement of slugs, but they won't do anything to actually repel them. The depth necessary for the eggshells to deter slugs would require breaking quite a few eggs to protect the typical garden, certainly more than would normally be produced in a day of baking. My best estimate would be a dozen eggs to create a $\frac{1}{4}$-inch deep ring that is 2 inches wide around a small plant. If you really want to repel slugs organically then take a look at diatomaceous earth, but be sure to use a diatomaceous earth product that is intended for use on slugs and insects rather than for swimming pools. The diatomaceous earth sold for use in swimming pool filters is generally not effective on garden pests.

Pruning tar and other wound coatings 🌱

Coating pruning cuts and other tree wounds with various products to reduce the likelihood of infection is a common practice that has been used by generations before us and will probably be carried on for many more. The practice dates back to at least the 18th century, when Forsyth's composition was recommended for tree injuries (Lodeman 1906). Since Forsyth's time a number of other coatings, some homemade and some commercial, have been suggested for tree wounds. It seems logical that coating a wound would prevent disease and insects from entering—but does it?

The practice

Over the years a number of different dressings have been recommended for tree wounds. Coal tar and lead paint are some of the earliest recommendations, and both were commonly used in the late 19th and early 20th centuries (Bailey 1927). Later, various other coatings were tried, including fungicides such as Bordeaux mixture (Hudler and Jensen-Tracy 2002). A number of newer coatings exist today, including shellac and artificial resins, though tar is still available.

The theory

Covering a tree wound with some sort of durable compound has long been suggested to protect the tree from diseases and insects. Additionally, because of the exclusion of pests, the wound is thought to heal more quickly.

The real story

Indeed, wound coatings have been used for many years, but even in the early 20th century scientists were questioning the value of these dressings (Peets 1925; Bailey 1927). Most recent studies on the effects of wound coatings demonstrate that they are not particularly useful for reducing discoloration or speeding wound closure. After dissecting over 400 wounds that were either untreated or treated with shellac, polyurethane, varnish, asphalt, various chemicals incorporated into lanolin, or other coatings, Alex Shigo, the best-known researcher to study the effects of sealing wounds, concluded that painting over wounds was a waste of time (1981). In all fairness to these products, some studies demonstrate that treating wounds with coatings is at least somewhat useful (Mercer 1979), but most researchers currently believe there is little benefit to wound coatings.

If a tree appears unsightly because of a wound, covering the wound is a good way to conceal it (Hudler and Jensen-Tracy 2002). Some research has even indicated that initial formation of woundwood (the wood that grows over a wound) may be stimulated by wound coatings (Marshall 1931), though the rapid initial formation is quickly followed by a more typical response.

Many extension services still recommend coating wounds on trees that are known to be particularly susceptible to certain diseases. Pruning tar is most commonly recommended for oak because of oak wilt, a terminal disease of oak, for elms because of Dutch elm disease, and for fruit trees such as apple and pear, where canker-causing bacteria and fungi create problems, fireblight being the most common. Evidence that wound coatings aid the tree in fighting off insects and disease, even in these extreme cases, is lacking. However, since the wound coating itself is unlikely to cause significant injury and since these diseases can be so devastating for the tree, it does seem reasonable to add pruning tar under these circumstances. Simply pruning these trees when they, and the diseases, are dormant would actually be a better way to deal with the diseases in most circumstances.

What it means to you

For most trees ❀❀. Sealing wounds for aesthetic purposes is a perfectly reasonable way to use these products. As a general rule, however, applying coatings to protect wounds is a practice that has not proved itself effective over the years, despite ample opportunity to do so.

For oaks, elms, and fruit trees ❀❀❀. In a few situations, applying a coating to wounds might be beneficial (beyond aesthetic reasons) and is certainly worth the risk. Oaks, elms, and fruit trees are vulnerable to a variety of diseases that can infect them through pruning wounds. In these cases the potential devastation may warrant the use of this treatment, although evidence of its effectiveness is wanting.

Tree wrap 🌱

Tree wraps in one form or another have been with us for a long time. Both white wash and wire structures were used for trees growing in city streets in the 19th century (Crozier 1888). Today, wrapping the base of a tree trunk with things like cardboard, commercially available plastic wraps, or wire is thought to prevent a variety of tree problems, including insect damage, rodent damage, and frost cracks. Frost cracks occur over the winter months, when sunlight is reflected off snow and onto the tree trunk. When the reflected light hits the trunk, the area that is being heated by the sun becomes physiologically active while the rest of the tree stays dormant, leading to bark splitting.

The practice

Many products have been recommended for wrapping trees. The most common are commercially available paper and plastic wraps, though home-made wraps are sometimes also suggested. Homemade wraps may include many different materials such as fiberglass insulation or even aluminum foil.

The theory

Tree wraps are supposed to serve as a barrier to such things as insects, rodents, and mowers, as well as to block reflected light from snow.

The real story

Tree wraps can repel certain boring insects that affect the trunk of trees, but they have also been reported to increase the incidence of insects in situations where the wrap is tightly applied: the insect actually lives in the space between the tree and the wrap (Owen et al. 1991). Wraps, especially those made of plastic, do seem to provide protection from physical damage caused by mowers, weed whackers, and even rodents, but they do not degrade rapidly, which can lead to problems. Bonnie Appleton, one of the leading researchers in tree wrap technology, recommended avoiding tree wraps because of potential long-term problems, but she also noted that a white polypropylene fabric might be an effective wrap because of its ability to degrade (1994), an important consideration because of people's propensity to forget about things.

If you forget about a tree wrap and it doesn't degrade, some serious effects could occur as the tree grows too large for the wrap. In fact, the biggest problems associated with applying tree wraps are girdling or constriction of the stem (Appleton and French 1992).

Tree wraps made from corrugated paper, commonly found in garden centers for use as winter protection, are not going to provide the same level of protection against mowers and other machinery that plastic wraps do; however, they will degrade. Though they are designed for winter protection these wraps do not seem to help protect trees from frost cracks to any great extent (Hart and Dennis 1978), and they are also unable to buffer temperatures near the trunk of the tree (Litzow and Pellett 1983). It is more likely that a lighter-colored material, one that is better able to reflect light than a corrugated paper tree wrap, would be more useful for protecting against frost cracks. Painting a tree trunk white has been suggested to serve this purpose (Relf and Appleton 2001).

What it means to you ❀❀❀

Tree wraps aren't a terrible idea, but not all trees need them. If you have few rodents around, and you're careful not to hit trees with your mower, then much of the common rationale for applying tree wraps is gone. If you have young, tender trees and are afraid of frost cracks, lightly colored tree wraps may benefit them by reflecting light. Care needs to be taken, however, to remove these wraps in a timely manner—they should be on the tree for no more than 6 months. If that doesn't seem possible, consider white washing the trunk of your tree. Large trees should not need to be wrapped because their bark should be thick enough to protect them from most animals and frost cracks.

Water mist for frost protection

Misting plants with water or turning a sprinkler on to keep plants wet when temperatures dip below freezing in the early spring has been suggested as a way to protect plants from frost. A jacket of ice can certainly be pretty, but is it really warm?

The practice

Sprinklers or misters are turned on to give cold-sensitive plants a constantly freezing layer of water during periods of frost. The water is turned off when the danger of freezing temperatures is gone.

The theory

Some people think ice provides insulation for the plant, some people think the water itself will keep the plants warm, and some people think the actual process of freezing gives off heat.

The real story

When water freezes it does give off heat, called "heat of fusion." This is something people learn in high school physics but forget soon afterward. The lesson didn't stick with me until I began to work with large nurseries. When there is a danger of a late frost nursery managers cannot place a protective cover over all their crops because it would take too long. Instead they put covers, such as polyethylene tarps, over their most valuable plants and turn on their sprinklers all night for everything else. As the water from the sprinklers hits the plants it freezes and that process actually helps to warm the plants.

Most research on how much protection can be achieved through the use of water sprays has been done with citrus fruit, where a frost can decimate a crop. This research has shown that protection during temperatures as low as 15 degrees Fahrenheit (–9 degrees Celsius) might be possible, at least for short periods of time (Braud et al. 1981).

What it means to you ❁❁❁

If your plants have started to grow in the early spring and a frost is imminent, applying water during the time that temperatures dip below freezing has a real chance of helping out your plants. Water application is not a miracle cure, and some plants can't handle frosts even when water is applied, but for most plants a real benefit is possible. Do be careful of drowning the plants you are trying to protect. If your soil is clay or is not well drained, you could possibly do more harm than good by applying irrigation all night. Also be aware that a light mist is all that is needed.

Putting it all together

In this chapter we took a look at a wide variety of products and practices that might prove useful, depending on your particular situation and the types of critters that you have to deal with. Some work and some don't. We've spent a long enough time looking at the practices and products that don't work, so let's not waste our time with those but instead consider the more promising options.

The best of the best

A few problem solvers are effective if done properly. Of these, my favorite is bagging fruit because it not only looks avant-garde, but it also actually works! Bagging fruit is a great idea for any home gardener who has found a maggot in their apple. Sure, it takes a lot of work, but the returns can be great. Spotless fruit is difficult to get in home gardens, even if you are willing to use pesticides. If you're not willing to use them, it can be downright impossible. Bags take care of most problems that commonly affect fruits, without the added dangers of pesticides. I think only one other practice is as useful as bagging fruit: beer traps for slugs.

Properly arranged beer traps are among the safest and most effective ways to get rid of slugs. Slugs are attracted to beer, and if the trap is properly oriented, slugs will fall into the beer and die, hopefully happier than if they were killed with a synthetic chemical. Beer traps are rarely dangerous to other critters, but it is probably best to make sure that local dogs and cats don't spend their time lapping it up. While beer is certainly not the beverage of choice for your dog or cat, it is much better for them than other slug killers, especially metaldehyde, a commercial slug and snail killer that is both toxic and somewhat attractive to many household pets. Although eggshells are supposed to be able to function as an effective slug barrier, I have seen no evidence of this. I'll stick with my beer traps.

The best of the rest

A few problem solvers in this chapter provide significant benefit, but not enough to get mentioned with the best of the best. These concoctions and practices are far from perfect, but depending on the situation, they are certainly worth trying. There are two practices that I have used and really like, though they have some significant drawbacks that may affect a person's decision to use them. The first is deer repellent, a great idea that sometimes works and sometimes doesn't.

Choosing plants that deer don't like is the best way to stay deer free, but homemade and commercial deer repellents are at least somewhat effective at keeping these four-legged pests off garden plants as long as there is a sufficient number of other plants nearby that the deer can eat.

DECIDUOUS TREES	DECIDUOUS SHRUBS	NEEDLE EVERGREENS	BROADLEAF EVERGREENS	PERENNIALS AND BULBS	ANNUALS
Birch	Butterfly bush	White fir	Glossy abelia	Bee balm	Ageratum
Dogwood	Summer sweet	Cedar	Azalea	Daffodil	Allium
Smokebush	Contoneaster	Douglas fir	Boxwood	Bleeding Heart	Coleus
Ginkgo	Forsythia	Juniper	Daphne	False indigo	Cosmos
Honeylocust	Cinquefoil	Larch	Hollies	Foxglove	Dahlia
Hawthorne	Japanese Rose	Spruce	Mahonia	Heath	Tobacco
Magnolia	Spiraea	Pine	Heavenly bamboo	Iris	Sage
Maple	St. John's Wort		Cherry laurel	Joe-pye weed	Snapdragon
Oak	Lilac		Fire thorn	Lamb's ear	Marigold
Red Elder	Arrow-wood		Arrow-wood	Lavender	Vervain
Sassafras	Weigela			Primula	Zinnia
				Sage	
				Speedwell	
				Spurge	
				Yarrow	

Figure 9. Common deer resistant plants that might prove more effective than deer repellents at reducing grazing, especially in the long run.

A second good idea with a few problems is tree wrap. Tree wrap, like deer repellent, is not foolproof, and tree wraps used incorrectly can cause severe damage to trees. However, tree wraps do provide protection from small animals, frost cracks, and weed whip–wielding teenagers. Although most professional arborists and horticulturists don't like to admit it, leaving a plastic spiral wrap on a tree for a few years will create a really neat-looking, contorted tree. It is unfortunate that this type of makeover is often terminal.

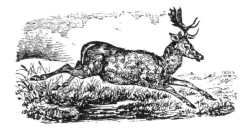

9

Commercial Pesticides

COMMERCIAL pesticides are used for killing (or in some cases repelling) insects, diseases, and weeds in your garden. Most of these chemicals have been around for a long time for use in other crops but have only relatively recently become available for homeowners.

Because of the nature of our world and the constant search for less toxic methods to control pests, the availability of various pesticides constantly changes. Paris green, London purple, and lead arsenate, which were the gold standard for controlling insect pests in the late 1800s and early 1900s, were overtaken by the safer and more effective pesticide DDT and the organophosphates in the 1940s and 1950s. DDT is now banned, and organophosphates probably won't be with us for too much longer. Looking through old pesticide books I often find myself thinking that our forefathers were crazy to use the potent poisons that they did. I wonder if, in another 100 years, our progeny will say the same thing about us.

How pesticides work

Though it is well beyond the scope of this book to address all the ways commercial pesticides can affect pests, it is useful to have a basic understanding of how the more-common ones work. If you are looking for more depth and would like a resource on the subject, *The Pesticide Book* by George Ware (2000) would be an excellent addition to your library.

Insecticides

In general, insecticides are more dangerous for humans than other types of pesticides (except those intended for use on mammals) because insects are more similar to humans than fungi, bacteria, and weeds are. Although insects and humans have organs that appear quite different, they function using the same basic principles.

Most commercial insecticides work by affecting the nervous system. These pesticides cause the insect's nerves to be stimulated, and they block the insect's ability to shut those nerve impulses off. This leads to extremely rapid death, which is the reason why the compounds are so popular; people like to see their target insect die rapidly, especially when they're dealing with wasps. Since humans also have nervous systems, most of these poisons can have some effect on humans, especially in large doses. In fact, some insecticides used today were discovered during research programs created to investigate nerve agents for killing people in World War II.

Commercial insecticides may also utilize stomach poisons such as the organic insecticide B.t., smothering agents such as oil, and growth regulators such as hydroprene. These poisons are usually safer for the applicator than nerve poisons, but should not be considered completely innocuous.

Fungicides

Fungicides generally work in one of two ways. The first is by inhibiting spore germination. When a fungal spore hits a leaf it germinates and grows into the tissue of the leaf. If a chemical is present on the leaf surface to inhibit this germination, the fungus cannot infect the plant. The second way a fungicide can work is by inhibiting the growth of the fungus after it germinates. In both cases the fungicide blocks the normal physiological processes of the pest to stop it from attacking the plant. Fungicides are, for the most part, the least understood of the three major pesticide classifications.

Herbicides

Herbicides work in a variety of ways, depending upon which ones you are applying. The most common herbicides used to kill non-grass weeds affect those weeds by mimicking natural auxins. These herbicides are actually quite similar to IBA and NAA and they affect non-grasses much more strongly than grasses. If applied at the proper concentration, they are very effective at killing weeds and preserving grass.

The most common synthetic auxins used as herbicides today include 2,4-D and its relatives. They work by confusing the plant. Since auxins occur naturally in the growing tips of plants and provide the plant with signals as to where to focus growth, the application of herbicides that mimics auxins will cause the plant to lose sight of where it should grow. This leads to curling, oddly shaped growth, and eventually death.

Another way that herbicides work is by inhibiting plants from creating basic chemicals that they need to live. Glyphosate is a commonly used herbicide that effectively kills most types of plants. It works by preventing the plant from creating a certain amino acid (protein). It does not kill the plant quickly but instead starves the plant to death by preventing it from constructing a necessary nutrient.

Herbicides that are intended to prevent weeds from sprouting, called preemergent herbicides, may work in a variety of ways. Prevention of seed germination is a common way that these chemicals work, but they may also affect the growth of the very young roots or shoots of the plant immediately after it emerges from the seed. The exact way that a young seed or plant is affected is not always completely understood, but in general, herbicides are better understood than fungicides.

Choosing a pesticide

When selecting a pesticide, consider three main factors. The first is safety. There is nothing more important than safety when applying any chemical. All pesticides are toxic to some extent, or they wouldn't control pests. Read the label before buying and before applying any compound. There is no substitute for reading and following the label. The second of the factors to consider is the residual. The residual of a compound indicates how long it will be effective at killing or repelling the target pest. Residuals of pesticides vary, depending on environmental conditions and the type of pesticide that is being applied. Herbicides with a long residual can last for many months, while a fungicide or insecticide with a long residual will rarely provide control for longer that a single month. The third factor that should be considered when deciding on a pesticide is selectivity. Pesticides often affect more than we intend. This can be good or bad. Controlling cabbage loopers and flea beetles at the same time is good. Killing beneficial insects, such as lady beetles, while trying to control caterpillars is bad. Herbicides and fungicides tend to be less selective than insecticides because people tend to want to control many types of weeds and many types of disease when they apply these compounds. Insecticides, on the other hand, run an amazing gamut of selectivity. Many insecticides target a wide variety of insects, but a number of insecticides target only a few specific organisms. In general, more-selective insecticides are safer for you, beneficial insects, and plants.

Figure 10 at the end of this chapter gives some information on a wide variety of chemicals that are, have recently been, or may soon be, available to the homeowner. If you think a compound looks useful, you should look for it in the active ingredient list on products available at your local garden center. Once you find a product that seems to have the traits you want, read the label and make sure that it is legal to use the pesticide in the way that you want to. Once again, there is no substitute for the label.

When reading the table, keep in mind that it lists the residual of the various active ingredients relative to other pesticides of the same type. In general, insecticides with a short residual will last less than 2 days, insecticides with a medium residual will last for about a week to 10 days, and insecticides with a long residual will usually last for more than 10 days. Fungicides with a short residual will typically last for less than a week, fungicides with a medium residual will last from 1 to 2 weeks, and fungicides with a long residual will last for more than 2 weeks. Herbicides with a short residual will generally last less than 1 week, herbicides with a medium residual will last from 1 week to 1 month, and herbicides with a long residual will last for over a month. Also remember that selectivity is very different between herbicides, fungicides, and insecticides because insecticides are often more specific than the other two types of pesticides.

The notes column indicates whether a compound is primarily a systemic or contact toxin. Insecticides and fungicides that are systemic will move throughout a plant and affect the disease or insect even if the spray itself does not contact the pest. Herbicides that are systemic will move throughout a plant's system, thereby effectively killing the plant at its roots. Contact insecticides and fungicides must somehow touch the disease or insect, or else they will have little effect. Contact herbicides will kill the portion of the plant that they touch but will not translocate to the root system, so there is a chance that the weed will resprout from the unaffected roots.

The notes on the herbicides indicate whether a chemical is a preemergent or postemergent compound. Preemergent compounds are intended to stop seeds from growing and have little effect on plants after they sprout from the ground. Postemergent compounds primarily affect plants after they sprout from the ground. Preemergent compounds tend to have much longer residuals that postemergent compounds.

Commercial pesticides work, and as long as you take the time to use them properly you will get reasonably good results. Generally, commercial pesticides are safe if proper care and handling guidelines, as outlined on the label, are followed.

ACTIVE INGREDIENT	RESIDUAL	SELECTIVITY	PESTICIDE TYPE AND OTHER NOTES
Insecticides			
Acephate	Medium	Kills many pests and is not as hard on beneficial insects as other synthetic insecticides are	Contact, with some systemic activity
Allethrin	Medium	Broad spectrum	Contact
Bacillus thuringiensis	Medium	May kill beetles, mosquitos, or caterpillars depending on the type of B.t. purchased	Organic. A stomach poison that must be ingested by the insect to work
Beauvaria bassiana	Long. Lives in soil or on plant.	Effective on many insects, including beetles	Organic. Contact. A fungus that feeds on insects. Very effective in high humidity conditions
Bifenthrin	Long	Effective on many insects and mites	Contact
Capsaicin	Short-Medium	Affects many insects	Works primarily as a repellant, keeping insects away rather than killing them. See the section on hot peppers for more information
Carbaryl	Medium	Effective on many insects but is most effective on beetles. Can devastate lady beetle populations	Contact poison. Replaced by permethrin for many household applications

Figure 10. A variety of pesticides and information relative to their use. Note that characteristics may vary depending upon the specific formulation used.

ACTIVE INGREDIENT	RESIDUAL	SELECTIVITY	PESTICIDE TYPE AND OTHER NOTES
Insecticides (continued)			
Cyfluthrin	Medium–Long	Effective on many different insects	Contact
Limonene	Short–Medium	Broad spectrum	A contact poison that comes from citrus peels. May damage plants
Deltamethrin	Medium–Long	Broad spectrum	Contact
Diatomaceous earth	Short–Medium	Effective on snails and some soft-bodied insects	Organic. This is a collection of once living organisms called diatoms, which are essentially small shards of "glass"
Diazinon	Long	Broad spectrum	Contact
Disulfoton/DiSyston	Long	Most effective on sucking insects such as aphids	Systemic. Should be used with extreme caution, as it is water soluble and very toxic
Esfenvalerate	Long	Broad spectrum	Contact. May take 3 days to kill but immediately stops insects from feeding
Hydroprene	Long	Most commonly applied for roaches, but does affect other insects	Contact. Alters the normal growth of insects and their reproductive ability but does not kill them outright
Imidacloprid	Long	Works best on aphids and leafminers. Not usually effective on mites and has been reported to increase mite populations	Systemic
Malathion	Short	Broad spectrum	Contact
Methoxychlor	Long	Broad spectrum	Contact. One of the last remaining and safest relatives of DDT
Milky spore disease (*Bacillus popillae*)	Long	Effective only on Japanese beetles	Organic. Contact. A bacterium that infects the Japanese beetle, usually killing it
Mint oil	Short	Broad spectrum	Organic. Contact
Neem	Medium	Broad spectrum	Organic. Contact. Derived from the Neem tree. One of the best botanical insecticides available. Also effective on some fungi
Oil	Medium	Effective primarily on soft bodied insects like aphids	Organic. Kills by smothering. Good coverage of plant material is especially important. May damage plants if misapplied

ACTIVE INGREDIENT	RESIDUAL	SELECTIVITY	PESTICIDE TYPE AND OTHER NOTES
Permethrin	Medium-Long	Broad spectrum	Contact. Has become one of the most common insecticides in recent years
Piperonyl butoxide	Short-Medium	Broad spectrum	Almost never used alone. Helps the activity of other insecticides
Pyrethrin	Short	Broad spectrum	Organic. Contact. Can be produced synthetically
Resmethrin	Short	Broad spectrum	Contact. Similar to pyrethrin
Rotenone	Medium	Broad spectrum	Organic. Very toxic to fish. One of the most toxic botanicals to humans. Derived from South American derris root. Extreme care should be taken with this product. I think this product would not be around if it weren't organic.
Soap	Short	Not effective on hard bodied pests	Organic. See the entry "Dish Soap" in chapter 5 for more information
Sodium laurel sulfate	Short	Broad spectrum	Organic. A type of soap
Spinosad	Medium	Effective on thrips, flies, and caterpillars. Does not kill most beneficials	Contact. May be organic depending on formulation
Tetramethrin	Short	Broad spectrum	Contact

Herbicides

ACTIVE INGREDIENT	RESIDUAL	SELECTIVITY	PESTICIDE TYPE AND OTHER NOTES
2,4-D	Short	Effective on broad leaf weeds such as dandelions	Postemergent. Systemic. Has been available since the 1940s. High temperatures make this compound damaging to grasses.
Acifluorfen	Short	Good for certain weeds. Read label	Postemergent. Contact. May harm many beneficial plants. Do not apply in hot, humid conditions
Calcium acid methanearsonate	Short	Effective on many annual weed grasses. Relatively safe for most turf grasses	Postemergent. Contact
Dicamba	Short	Effective on most broadleaf weeds. Dangerous for trees— use with care	Postemergent. Systemic
Diquat	Short	Broad spectrum	Postemergent. Contact herbicide that acts quickly and is very effective on most weeds

ACTIVE INGREDIENT	RESIDUAL	SELECTIVITY	PESTICIDE TYPE AND OTHER NOTES
Herbicides (continued)			
Dithiopyr	Long	Broad spectrum	Preemergent, with some postemergent properties
Garlic oil	Short	Effective on most weeds, but perennials may resprout	Organic. Postemergent. Contact. May not affect roots
Glufosinate-ammonium	Short	Broad spectrum	Postemergent. Contact, with some systemic activity. Fast acting
Glyphosate	Short	Broad spectrum. Not particularly effective on thistle or horsetail	Postemergent. Systemic. Most widely used broad spectrum product available. Takes a long time to work, often a week or more
Mecoprop (MCPP)	Short	Effective on broad leaf weeds	Postemergent. Systemic. Takes a long time to kill weeds, often a week or more
Monosodium acid methanearsonate (MSMA)	Short	Effective on many annual grasses. Relatively safe for most turf grasses	Postemergent. Contact
Oxyfluorfen	Long	Effective on most weeds, depending on the concentration applied	Preemergent
Pelargonic acid	Short	Broad spectrum	Postemergent. Contact
Siduron	Medium	Does not affect the seeds of most cool season grasses (such as Kentucky bluegrass and fescues), but does affect the seeds of many weeds	Preemergent
Triclopyr	Short	Primarily for broad leaf weeds, but damages grass if over-applied. Often used for woody vines	Postemergent. Systemic. Some pesticides with this active ingredient can be used near turf, but care must be taken not to overapply.
Trifluralin	Long	Broad spectrum	Preemergent
Disease Control			
Bonomyl (thiophanate-methyl)	Long	Broad spectrum	Systemic
Bordeaux mixture	Medium	Broad spectrum	Organic. Contact. Produces an ugly, milky blue-green coating on surfaces to which it is applied. One of the oldest fungicides still available, it was discovered in the

ACTIVE INGREDIENT	RESIDUAL	SELECTIVITY	PESTICIDE TYPE AND OTHER NOTES
			1860s when it was applied to deter people from eating wine grapes in the Bordeaux region of France. Those grapes were the only ones that survived a severe outbreak of downy mildew.
Captan	Medium	Broad spectrum	Contact. May injure fruits, including apples and pears
Chlorothalonil	Medium	Broad spectrum	Contact. May cause golden apples to discolor
Copper	Medium	Broad spectrum	Organic. Contact
Mancozeb	Medium	Broad spectrum	Contact
Potassium bicarbonate	Short–Medium	Broad spectrum	Organic. Contact. Similar to baking soda
Propiconazole	Medium–Long	Broad spectrum. Some reports indicate efficacy on blackspot is marginal	Systemic
Streptomycin	Short–Medium	Broad spectrum bactericide. Not a fungicide. Most commonly used for fireblight. Some resistance is present.	Contact
Sulfur	Short–Medium	Broad spectrum	Organic. Contact. Smells bad
Thiram	Medium	Broad spectrum	Contact
Triadimefon	Medium–Long	Broad spectrum	Systemic
Triforine	Medium	Broad spectrum. Usually effective on blackspot. Good for powdery mildew	Systemic

Others

ACTIVE INGREDIENT	RESIDUAL	SELECTIVITY	PESTICIDE TYPE AND OTHER NOTES
Cytokinin	_____	Works on many plants	This hormone increases the size of cells in plants. It works better on some plants than others. Read the label carefully.
Ethephon	_____	Works on many plants	A plant hormone that causes fruit to drop prematurely
Gibberellic acid	_____	Works well on some plants but not others	A plant hormone that tricks the plant into thinking it has been fertilized. Will provide superior fruit set in some plants. Does not always work well. Timing must be good, or it will fail.

ACTIVE INGREDIENT	RESIDUAL	SELECTIVITY	PESTICIDE TYPE AND OTHER NOTES
Others (continued)			
Iron phosphate	A week or longer	Effective on slugs and snails but not insects	Organic. A slug and snail killer
Metaldehyde	A week or longer	Effective on slugs and snails but not insects	A slug and snail killer. Has the potential to harm some pets, especially dogs
Warfarin	Used as a bait, this chemical can last quite a long time	Effective on rats, mice, and other rodents	A rodenticide usually used as a bait

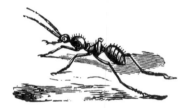

10

Concoctions to be Avoided

Before you picked up this book you probably realized that some practices recommended for gardeners are questionable. Some questionable practices, however, are worse than others. This chapter won't deal with practices that might or might not work, but rather with those practices that are guaranteed to make a mess of things. For example, while I would hesitate to tell a home gardener not to try hydrogels, as there is some evidence out there that they might work and little evidence that they would do any extensive damage to your plants, I would strongly discourage them from using hydrocyanic acid gas to kill insects, something that is recommended in *A Little Book of Climbing Plants* published in 1933. (The author, A. Hottes, does encourage a "hasty exit" after the cyanide gas is released.) This chapter pays homage to the worst of the worst. Without further ado, here are what I personally consider to be the five worst recommendations for the home gardener.

A crazy old remedy

This first mix is from a book by Ernst Lodeman titled *The Spraying of Plants* (1906), the first edition of which came out in 1896. In this book the author delivered a rich and wonderful history of pesticide application based on his examination of old European and American recipes for pesticides. One crazy remedy he found, while not to my knowledge used today, should never have been in use. The fact that it ever was says a great deal about people's knowledge of controlling plant disease. As Lodeman states, this mixture "contained some materials which unquestionably possessed 'strength' but whether best adapted for the purpose designed may be open to doubt." The mix, recommended in 1849, was intended to provide a cure for mildew on peaches with a single application made in April.

The mix

One hectoliter (26.4 gallons) of urine was added to 25 liters (6.6 gallons) of pigeon dung and allowed to ferment for 48 hours, at which point 1 kilogram (2.2 pounds) of aconite branches (a plant also known as monk's hood) was added, along with 4 liters (3.8 gallons) of water. This mix was then applied to leaves to destroy mildew.

Why this recipe is a bad idea

This recipe actually may work; after all, adding water to the leaves of plants may inhibit powdery mildew by itself. The main reason to avoid this mixture is not that it won't work but that it is dangerous for people to apply pigeon dung on things that humans eat. Besides, it is downright disgusting.

Conclusion

Even if you could find 25 liters of pigeon dung, it would be a bad idea to apply this concoction because of its potential effect on human health. I can't see this concentration of dung and urine being particularly healthy for plant foliage, either.

A confusion of pH

This next mix is one that I have seen in various home-gardening books and on the Web. It is intended to cure yellowing in shrubs and trees, usually azaleas and rhododendrons.

The mix

Lime and some form of chelate, usually liquid iron, are mixed together. In various recipes other additions are included, but the lime and the chelate mixture is the important part.

Why this recipe is a bad idea

This mix includes one ingredient that is probably useful and one that is so bad it will actually hurt your plant. Azaleas and rhododendrons commonly turn yellow because their soil is too alkaline (the pH is too high). When the pH is too high, iron is not available to the plant, and the plant suffers. The iron chelate in the above recipe will help the shrub if high pH is the problem, but the lime will actually increase the pH of the soil and could very possibly burn any foliage it touches. If you apply this mixture the plant will probably perk up because of the chelated iron and then go downhill after 2 or 3 months because of the lime.

Conclusion

Do not use this recipe ever. I can think of no circumstance where it will help and in most cases it will actually make the problem worse.

Burn, baby, burn

Using ammonia from your cleaning cabinet as a fertilizer is, as we have already seen, not a particularly good idea. However, some methods of using this cleaner are worse than others.

The mix

Common recommendations suggest filling more than half of the reservoir of a hose-end sprayer with ammonia.

Why this recipe is a bad idea

The problem with this recipe is that the ammonia is much too concentrated to be applied to a lawn, especially in the hot summer. This mixture is likely to scorch grass. I first saw the recipe used in Florida, and in early spring in Florida, where sandy soils might allow the ammonia to move through the ground quickly, you might get away without much damage. In most locations, however, this stuff is a good way to burn your lawn.

Conclusion

This mixture is likely to cause a great deal of damage to a lawn.

Hitchhikers in the tobacco

Tobacco can be effective for those determined to produce their own insecticides. However, this plant can produce some unwanted side effects when mixed in a solution to kill insects.

The mix

Chewing tobacco products are mixed into an insecticidal spray for getting rid of insects on tomatoes; the most common target is hornworms.

Why this recipe is a bad idea

Tobacco plants and tomato plants share many diseases, such as tobacco mosaic virus and tomato spotted wilt virus. The curing process for tobacco will not necessarily get rid of these diseases. By applying an insecticidal mixture that contains tobacco juice, you may actually expose your tomato plant to a disease more damaging than the insects you are trying to kill.

Conclusion

To avoid trading an insect problem for a disease problem, do not apply any form of tobacco to your tomatoes.

This will do the job (and more)

Commercial pesticides can be, and often are, incorrectly used. If you deviate from labeled recommendations you can cause severe problems for your plants or yourself. Here is an older recommendation that some people periodically try with devastating results.

The mix

Glyphosate is sometimes recommended to get rid of tree suckers (small shoots that emerge near the base of the tree).

Why this recipe is a bad idea

Glyphosate is a systemic herbicide. It actually moves from the leaf surface to the roots of the plant. Since the tree's suckers and the tree itself share a common root system, it is likely that any systemic herbicide sprayed onto the tree's suckers will affect the health of the tree, perhaps even killing it.

Conclusion

Don't apply any form of systemic herbicide, especially glyphosate, to tree suckers. To take it one step further, never use any pesticide in a manner contrary to the instructions listed on the label; it is stupid and dangerous to do so. If a pesticide doesn't have a label, don't buy it or use it.

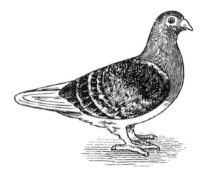

11

Take Home Message

EVEN IF YOU don't remember what I've written about deer repellents, beer, tobacco, or baking soda, remember this take home message: Search for the *why* behind everything you do for your plants. Do not settle for unexplained recommendations.

We have seen all kinds of different techniques for treating plants, from buttermilk to beer, from sound to soda. Some techniques look pretty good, some look pretty bad, and some look just plain silly, but the information offered here isn't the end of the story, not by a long shot. In fact, I hope this is only the beginning for you, a start on the road to understanding the many techniques available for growing your plants. I have enjoyed going through the old books, finding the recent articles, and especially doing the experiments needed to get to the facts behind the recommendations and products, but the last thing I want you to do is to take my word for it. Challenge my findings. Don't be satisfied with the depth of my answers, look deeper into the literature, read the old gardening guides, a category that will one day include this book. And experiment. Get ten *Pachysandra*, treat five with buttermilk, and leave five alone. Take twelve Peonies and play Mozart for four, Led Zepplin for four more, and leave the last four alone in blissful peace. Open a bottle of beer and fertilize some weeds. (I really don't think that you should give beer to any plant that you prize.) Maybe I tried the wrong beer, maybe a nice California microbrew like Anchor Porter will do the job that Michelob, Sharps, and Guinness couldn't. Divide off a section of plants in your garden just for experimenting and have fun with them. Yes, that means some might be damaged, but it also means that the plants you buy in the future will be cared for by a more thoughtful and educated person. There will be successes and failures, but with each new experiment you will be a wiser gardener. One final word on experimenting: be careful. Many home-brewed pesticides and fertilizers have drawbacks that need to be thoroughly investigated before you try them. Additionally, experimenting with pesticides outside of labeled recommendations can be dangerous for you and your plants. Don't do it.

Working with plants is fun. We garden because it relaxes us, educates us, lets us commune with nature, and, above all, makes us feel good. Enjoy your trees, enjoy your garden, and let them be a part of your life. And again, search for the *why* behind everything that you do for your plants. Do not settle for unexplained recommendations. Your plants deserve more and so do you.

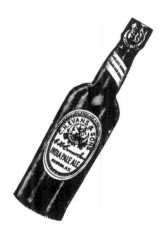

APPENDIX 1

Preferred pH of Some Common Landscape Plants

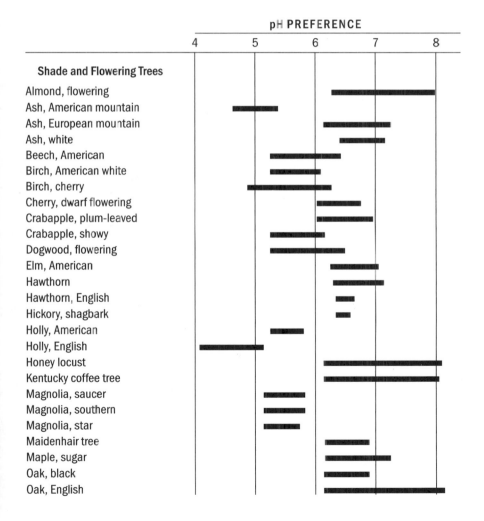

pH PREFERENCE

	4	5	6	7	8

Shade and Flowering Trees

- Almond, flowering
- Ash, American mountain
- Ash, European mountain
- Ash, white
- Beech, American
- Birch, American white
- Birch, cherry
- Cherry, dwarf flowering
- Crabapple, plum-leaved
- Crabapple, showy
- Dogwood, flowering
- Elm, American
- Hawthorn
- Hawthorn, English
- Hickory, shagbark
- Holly, American
- Holly, English
- Honey locust
- Kentucky coffee tree
- Magnolia, saucer
- Magnolia, southern
- Magnolia, star
- Maidenhair tree
- Maple, sugar
- Oak, black
- Oak, English

pH PREFERENCE

	4	5	6	7	8

Shade and Flowering Trees
(continued)

Plant	pH Preference
Oak, pin	4.5–5.5
Oak, bur	7.8–8
Oak, red	4.5–5
Oak, southern live	5–5.5
Oak, white	6–7
Pecan	6–8
Sour gum	6–6.5
Sourwood	5.5–6
Sweet gum	6–6.5
Sycamore, American	6–7
Tulip tree	6–6.5
Willow, weeping	5–5.5
Witch hazel	6–7

Ornamental Shrubs

Plant	pH Preference
Azalea, hiryu	4.5–5.5
Azalea, pink	4–5
Barberry, Japanese	6–7
Bayberry	5–5.5
Beautybush	6–7
Boxwood, common	6–7
Butterfly bush	6–7
Buttonbush	6–8
Chokeberry, black	5–6
Chokeberry, red	5–5.5
Cotoneaster	6–8
Cotoneaster, rock	6.5–7
Daphne, February	6.5–7
Daphne, rose	6.5–7
Deutzia	6–7
Deutzia, Lemoine	6–8
Dogwood, goldentwig	6–7
Euonymus, winged	5.5–6.5
Fire thorn	6–8
Fringe tree, white	5–6
Hackberry, nettle tree	6–8
Heather, Scotch	4.5–5.5
Hibiscus, Chinese	6–8
Holly, Japanese	5.5–6
Hollygrape, Oregon	6–8

pH PREFERENCE

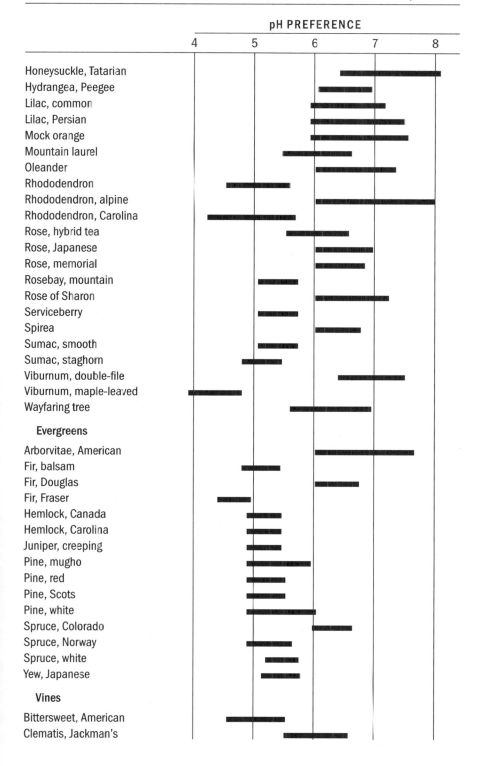

	4	5	6	7	8

Honeysuckle, Tatarian

Hydrangea, Peegee

Lilac, common

Lilac, Persian

Mock orange

Mountain laurel

Oleander

Rhododendron

Rhododendron, alpine

Rhododendron, Carolina

Rose, hybrid tea

Rose, Japanese

Rose, memorial

Rosebay, mountain

Rose of Sharon

Serviceberry

Spirea

Sumac, smooth

Sumac, staghorn

Viburnum, double-file

Viburnum, maple-leaved

Wayfaring tree

Evergreens

Arborvitae, American

Fir, balsam

Fir, Douglas

Fir, Fraser

Hemlock, Canada

Hemlock, Carolina

Juniper, creeping

Pine, mugho

Pine, red

Pine, Scots

Pine, white

Spruce, Colorado

Spruce, Norway

Spruce, white

Yew, Japanese

Vines

Bittersweet, American

Clematis, Jackman's

pH PREFERENCE

	4	5	6	7	8

Vines (continued)

Dutchman's pipe
Honeysuckle, trumpet
Ivy, Boston
Ivy, English
Virgin's bower
Wisteria, Japanese

Fruit Plants

Apple, common
Apricot
Blueberry, high bush
Cherry, sweet
Grapefruit
Orange, sweet
Peach
Pear, common
Plum, American
Raspberry, black
Raspberry, red

Grass

Bluegrass, annual
Bluegrass, Canada
Bluegrass, Kentucky
Fescue, chewing
Fescue, red

Ground Covers

Bearberry, common
Bugleweed, carpet

Source: C. H. Spurway 1944. Courtesy of Michigan State College Agricultural Experiment Station

APPENDIX 2

Conversion Tables

To convert length:	Multiply by:
Yards to meters	0.9
Inches to centimeters	2.54
Inches to millimeters	25.4
Feet to centimeters	30.5
Meters to yards	1.09
Meters to inches	39.4
Centimeters to inches	0.39
Millimeters to inches	0.04

To convert weight:	Multiply by:
Pounds to grams	453.59
Pounds to kilograms	2.2
Ounces to grams	28.35
Ounces to kilograms	0.028
Kilograms to pounds	0.455
Kilograms to ounces	35.274
Grams to pounds	.002
Grams to ounces	0.035

To convert area:	Multiply by:
Square inches to square centimeters	6.45
Square feet to square meters	0.093
Square yards to square meters	0.836
Acres to square meters	4046.8
Square centimeters to square inches	0.155
Square meters to square feet	10.8
Square meters to square yards	1.2

To convert volume:	Multiply by:
Gallons to liters	3.785
Teaspoons to milliliters	4.929
Tablespoons to milliliters	14.787
Pints to liters	0.473
Liters to gallons	0.264
Liters to pints	2.113
Milliliters to teaspoons	0.203
Milliliters to tablespoons	0.068

Bibliography

Adani, F., P. Genevini, P. Zaccheo, and G. Zocchi. 1998. The efficacy of commercial humic acid on tomato plant growth and mineral nutrition. *Journal of Plant Nutrition* 21: 561–575.

Alam, S., H. S. M. Imamul, S. Kawai, and A. Islam. 2002. Effects of applying calcium salts to coastal saline soils on   growth and mineral nutrition of rice varieties. *Journal of Plant Nutrition* 25: 561–576.

Al-Dahmani, J. H., P. A. Abbasi, S. A. Miller, and H. A. J. Hoitink. 2003. Suppression of bacterial spot of tomato with foliar sprays of compost extracts under greenhouse and field conditions. *Plant Disease* 87: 913–919.

Al-Khatib, K., C. Libbey, and R. Boydston. 1997. Weed suppression with *Brassica* green manure crops in green pea. *Weed Science* 45: 439–445.

Amonkar, S. V., and E. L. Reeves. 1970. Mosquito control with active principle of garlic, *Allium sativum*. *Journal of Economic Entomology* 63: 1172–1175.

Aoun, M. F., K. B. Perry., W. H. Swallow, D. J. Werner, and M. L. Parker. 1993. Antitranspirants and Cryoprotectants do not prevent peach freezing injury. *HortScience* 28: 343.

Appleton, B. L. 1994. Use and misuse of tree trunk protective wraps, paints and guards. Forestry Report R8-FR 44.

Appleton, B. L., and S. French. 1992. Current attitudes toward and uses of tree trunk protective wraps, paints and devices. *Journal of Arboriculture* 18: 15–20.

Arena, M. J., O. J. Schwarz, and W. T. Witte. 1997. Influence of black locust and contorted willow water diffusate on rooting stem cuttings. *Proceedings SNA Research Conference* 42: 20–22.

Back, E. A., and Pemberton, C. E., 1915. Susceptibility of citrus fruits to the attack of the Mediterranean fruit fly. *Journal of Agricultural Research* 3: 311–330.

Bahe, A. R., and C. H. Peacock. 1995. Bioavailable herbicide residues in turf-grass clippings used for mulch adversely affect plant growth. *HortScience* 30: 1393–1395.

Bailey, L. H. 1915. *The Standard Cyclopedia of Horticulture*. New York: Macmillan.

———. 1927. *The Pruning Manual*. New York: Macmillan.

Banuls, J., A. Quinones, B. Martin, E. Primo-Millo, and F. Legaz. 2003. Effects of the frequency of iron chelate supply by fertigation on iron chlorosis in citrus. *Journal of Plant Nutrition* 26: 1985–1996.

Bauder, J. W., and T. A. Brock. 2001. Irrigation water quality, soil amendment, and crop effects on sodium leaching. *Arid Land Research and Management* 15: 101–113.

Begna, S. H., L. M. Dwyer, D. Cloutier, L. Assemat, A. DiTommaso, X. Zhou, B. Prithiviraj, and D. L. Smith. 2002. Decoupling of light intensity effects on the growth and development of C3 and C4 weed species through sucrose supplementation. *Journal of Experimental Botany* 53: 1935–1940.

Bennett, A. C., and F. Adams. 1970. Concentration of NH_3 (aq) required for incipient NH_3 toxicity to seedlings. *Soil Science Society of America Proceedings* 34: 259–263.

Bilderback, T. E., M. R. Lorscheider, and R. U. Roeber. 1997. Wetting agents used in container substrates: are they BMP's? *Acta Horticulturae* 450: 313–319.

Bingaman, B. R., and N. E. Christians. 1995. Greenhouse screening of corn gluten meal as a natural control product for broadleaf and grass weeds. *HortScience* 30: 1256–1259.

Boatright, J. L., D. E. Balint, W. A. Mackay, and J.M. Zajicek. 1997. Incorporation of a hydrophilic polymer into annual landscape beds. *Journal of Environmental Horticulture* 15: 37–40.

Bonner, J., and F. Addicott. 1937. Cultivation of excised pea roots. *Botanical Gazette* 99: 144–170.

Bonner, J., and J. Greene. 1938. Vitamin B1 and the growth of green plants. *Botanical Gazette* 100: 226–237.

Bowen, P., J. Menzies, D. Ehret, L. Samuels, and A. D. M. Glass. 1992. Soluble silicon sprays inhibit powdery mildew development on grape leaves. *Journal of the American Society for Horticultural Science* 117: 906–912.

Braman, S. K., and J. G. Latimer. 2002. Effects of cultivar and insecticide choice on oleander aphid management and arthropod dynamics on *Asclepias* species. *Journal of Environmental Horticulture*. 20: 11–15.

Braud, H. J., P. Davidson, and P. L. Hawthorne. 1981. Reduction of freeze loss in citrus with water spray. *Transactions of the ASAE* 24: 396–400.

Broschat, T. K., and K A. Klock-Moore. 2000. Root and shoot growth responses to phosphate fertilization in container-grown plants. *Hort-Technology* 10: 765–767.

Brown, P. D., and M. J. Morra. 1995. Glucosinolate-containing plant tissues as bioherbicides. *Journal of Agricultural and Food Chemistry* 43: 3070–3074.

Buta, J. G., D. W. Spaulding, and A. N. Reed. 1987. Differential growth responses of fractionated turfgrass seed leachates. *HortScience* 22: 1317–1319.

Buwalda, J. G., and K. M. Goh. 1982. Host fungus competition for carbon as a cause of growth depression in vesicular arbuscular mycorrhizal ryegrass. *Soil Biology and Biochemistry* 14: 103–106.

Byun, H. J., and S. J. Choi. 2003. Suppression of post-harvest grey mold rot incidence in strawberry by field application of hydrogen peroxide. *Journal of the Korean Society for Horticultural Science* 44: 859–862.

Carlson, D. R. 1989. Process for Treating Plants. US Patent 4,834,789, filed Jul. 21, 1987, and issued May 30, 1989.

———. 1991. Process for Treating Plants. US Patent 5,043,009, filed May 26, 1989, and issued Aug. 27, 1991.

Carter, J. E., and R. R. Tripepi. 1989. Lifting date influences the ability of auxins to promote root regeneration of Colorado spruce. *Journal of Environmental Horticulture* 7: 147–150.

Catar, G. 1954. Effects of plant extracts on *Ixodes ricinus*. *Bratislava Medical News* 34: 1004–1010.

Ceulemans, R., R. Gabriels, and I. Impens. 1983. Antitranspirants effects on transpiration, net CO_2 exchange rate and water-use efficiency of azalea *Rhododendron simsii*. *Scientia Horticulturae* 19: 125–131.

Cherif, M., J. G. Menzies, D. L. Ehret, C. Bogdanoff, and R. R. Belanger. 1994. Yield of cucumber infected with *Pythium aphanidermatum* when grown with soluble silicon. *HortScience* 29: 896–897.

Christians, N. E. 1991. Preemergence Weed Control Using Corn Gluten Meal. US Patent 5,030,268, filed Jan. 16, 1990, and issued Jul. 9, 1991.

———. 1998. *Fundamentals of Turfgrass Management*. Chelsea, MI: Ann Arbor Press.

Cloyd, R. A., and N. L. Cycholl. 2002. Phytotoxicity of selected insecticides on greenhouse-grown herbs. *HortScience* 37: 671–672.

Columella, L. J. M. 1745. *Of husbandry. In twelve books; and his book concerning trees.* Trans. A. Millar. London: Andrew Millar Publisher.

Conover, D. L. 1987. Comparison of two repellents for reducing deer damage to Japanese yews during winter. Wildlife Society Bulletin 15: 265–268

Consumer Reports. 1998. When Bambi eats your flowers. 63(10): 32–33.

Cowles, R. S., J. E. Keller, and J. R. Miller. 1989. Pungent spices, ground red pepper, and synthetic capsaicin as onion fly ovipositional deterrents. *Journal of Chemical Ecology* 15: 719–730.

Cronin, M. J., D. S. Yohalem, R. F. Harris, and J. H. Andrews. 1996. Putative mechanisms and dynamics of inhibition of the apple scab pathogen *Venturia inaequalis* by compost extracts. Soil Biology and Biochemistry 28: 1241–1249.

Crouch, I. J., M. T. Smith, J. Van Staden, M. J. Lewis, and G. V. Hoad. 1992. Identification of auxins in a commercial seaweed concentrate. *Journal of Plant Physiology* 139: 590–594.

Crozier, A. A. 1888. Wire netting for tree guards. *Garden and Forest.* 1: 7.

Currey, J. A. 1924. Bicarbonate of soda spray effective. *The American Rose Annual* 9: 69–70.

Davidson, H., R. Mecklenberg, and C. Peterson. 2000. *Nursery Management.* Upper Saddle River, NJ: Prentice Hall.

Davy, H. 1814. *Elements of Agricultural Chemistry.* London: Longman, Hurst, Rees, Orme, and Brown.

deFeo, V., F. DeSimpne, F. Giannattasio, V. Magnifico, A. Marcantonio, and A. D. Palumbo. 1997. Allelopathic effects of broccoli extracts on vegetable crops. *Allelopathy Journal* 4: 277–281.

De Kreij, C., and H. Basar. 1995. Effect of humic substances in nutrient film technique on nutrient uptake. *Journal of Plant Nutrition* 18: 793–802.

deNardo, E. A. B., and P. S. Grewal. 2003. Compatibility of *Steinernema feltiae* with pesticides and plant growth regulators used in glasshouse plant production. *Biocontrol Science and Technology* 13: 441–448.

Dirr, M. A., and C. W. Heuser. 1987. *The Reference Manual of Woody Plant Propagation.* Varsity Press. Athens, GA.

Dole, J. M., and H. F. Wilkins. 1999. *Floriculture.* Upper Saddle River, NJ: Prentice Hall.

Dowie, E., and J. M. Oxley. 1899. Composition for Expelling Rats. US Patent 631,738.

du Toit L. J., and M. L. Derie. 2005. Evaluation of Actigard, bactericides, and compost teas for control of bacterial blight in carrot seed crops, 2004. *Fungicide and Nematicide Tests* 60: V046.

Elliot, M. L., and M. Prevatte. 1996. Response of 'Tifdwarf' Bermudagrass to seaweed derived biostimulants. *HortTechnology* 6: 261–263.

Englert, J. M., K. Warren, L. H. Fuchigami, and T. H. H. Chen. 1993. Anti-dessicant compounds improve the survival of bare-root deciduous nursery trees. *Journal of the American Society for Horticultural Science* 118: 228–235.

Fechner, G. T. 1909. *Nanna Oder uber das Seelenleben der Pflanzen*. Liepzig: L. Voss. (Orig. pub. 1848.)

Filer, T. H., and E. A. Nelson. 1987. Chemical treatments increase first year height growth and reduce dieback in cold storage sycamore (*Platanus occidentalis* L.) seedlings. *Tree Planters' Notes* 38: 26–30.

Fitzpatrick, M. S., C. B. Schreck, R. L. Chitwood, and L. L. Marking. 1995. Evaluation of three candidate fungicides for treatment of adult spring Chinook salmon. *Progressive Fish Culturist* 57: 153–155.

Flint, H. M., N. J. Parks, J. E. Holmes, J. A. Jones, and C. M. Higuera. 1995. Tests of garlic oil for control of the silverleaf whitefly, *Bemesia argentifollii* Bellows and Perring, in cotton. *Southwestern Entomological Society* 20: 137–150.

Fournier, V., and J. Brodeur. 2000. Dose-response susceptibility of pest aphids (Homoptera: Aphididae) and their control on hydroponically grown lettuce with the entomopathogenic fungus *Verticillium lecanii*, azadirachtin, and insecticidal soap. *Environmental Entomology* 29: 568–578.

Gardner, F. E. 1929. The relationship between tree age and the rooting of cuttings. *Proceedings of the American Society for Horticultural Science* 26: 101–104.

Gillman, J. H. 2004. Hydrogel amendments do not decrease the time interval between waterings for container-grown geranium or ninebark. *HortScience* 39: 820.

Gillman, J. H., and D. C. Zlesak. 2000. Applications of sodium silicate to rose (*Rosa* 'Nearly Wild') cuttings decreases leaflet drop and increases rooting. *HortScience* 35: 773.

Gillman, J. H., D. C. Zlesak, and J. A. Smith. 2003. Applications of potassium silicate decrease black spot infection in *Rosa hybrida* 'Meipelta'(Fuchsia Meidiland™). *HortScience* 38: 1144–1147.

Gillman, J. H., M. A. Dirr, and S. K. Braman. 1998. Effects of dolomitic lime on growth and nutrient uptake of *Buddleia davidii* 'Royal Red' grown in pine bark. *Journal of Environmental Horticulture* 16: 111–113.

Girourd, R. M., and C. E. Hess. 1964. The diffusion of root-promoting sub-
    stances from stems of *Hedera helix*. *Combined Proceedings of the International
    Plant Propagators Society* 14: 162–166.

Girth, H. B., E. E. McCoy, and R. W. Glaser. 1940. Field experiments with a
    nematode parasite of the Japanese beetle. New Jersey Agricultural Circu-
    lar 317.

Glaser, R. W. 1931. The cultivation of a nematode parasite of an insect. *Sci-
    ence* 73: 614–615.

Gorinstein, S., M. Zemser, F. Vargas-Albores, J. L. Ochoa, O. Paredes-
    Lopez, C. Scheler, J. Salnikow, O. Martin-Belloso, and S. Trakhtenberg.
    1999. Proteins and amino acids in beers, their contents and relationships
    with other analytical data. *Food Chemistry* 67: 71–78.

Gupta, P., and M. R. Siddiqui, 1999. Compatibility studies on *Steinernema
    carpocapsae* with some pesticidal chemicals. *Indian Journal of Entomology*
    61: 220–225.

Haggag, W. M. 2002. Application of epidermal coating antitranspirants for
    controlling cucumber downy mildew in greenhouse. Plant Pathology
    Bulletin 11: 69–78.

Hale, A. G. 1871. Stimulant for flowers. *The Horticulturist* 26: 165.

Hamner, C. L. 1940. Effects of vitamin B1 upon the development of some
    flowering plants. *Botanical Gazette*. 102: 156–168.

Hart, J. H., and G. K. Dennis. 1978. Effect of tree wrap on the incidence of
    frost crack in Norway maple. *Journal of Arboriculture* 4: 226–227.

Hartley, M. J., and A. Rahman. 1997. Organic mulches for weed control in
    apple orchards. *Orchardist* 70: 28–30.

Hedau, N. K., and M. Kumar. 2002. Effect of different mulches on yield,
    plant height, nitrogen uptake, weed control, soil moisture and economics
    of tomato cultivation. *Progressive Horticulture* 34: 208–210.

Henderson, P. 1890. *Handbook of Plants and General Horticulture*. New York:
    Peter Henderson.

Herrett, R. A., and P. A. King. 1967. Plant Growth Medium. US Patent
    3,336,129, filed Mar. 22, 1963, and issued Aug. 15, 1967.

Hess, C. E. 1959. A study of plant growth substances in easy and difficult to
    root cuttings. *Combined Proceedings of the International Plant Propagators
    Society* 9: 39–43.

Higgins, C. J. 1992. Western flower thrips in greenhouses: population
    dynamics, distribution on plants, and associations with predators. *Journal
    of Economic Entomology* 85: 1891–1903.

Hori, M. 1996. Settling inhibition and insecticidal activity of garlic and onion oils against *Myzus persicae* (Suzler). *Applied Entomology and Zoology* 31: 605–612.

Hottes, A. C. 1933. *A Little Book of Climbing Plants*. New York: A. T. De La Mare.

Huang, Y., S. X. Chen, and S. H. Ho. 2000. Bioactivities of methyl allyl disulfide and diallyl trisulfide from essential oil of garlic to two species of stored-product pests, *Sitophilus zeamais* and *Tribolium castaneum*. *Journal of Economic Entomology* 93: 537–543.

Hudler, G. W., and S. Jensen-Tracy. 2002. Lac Balsam as a treatment to hasten wound closure and minimize discoloration and decay. *Journal of Arboriculture* 28: 264–269.

Ibrahim, M. A., P. Kainulainen, A. Aflatuni, K. Tiilikkala, and J. K. Holopainen. 2001. Insecticidal, repellent, antimicrobial activity and phytotoxicity of essential oils: with special reference to limonene and its suitability for control of insect pests. *Agricultural and Food Science in Finland* 10: 243–259.

Ingham, E. 2000. *The Compost Tea Brewing Manual*. Corvalis, OR: Soil Foodweb.

Inglis, D. A., B. Gundersen, R. Houghton, and A. Kutz-Troutman. 2004. Evaluation of fungicides, compost tea, and host resistance for control of late blight on tomato, 2003. *Fungicide and Nematicide Tests* 59: V076.

Jing, C.S. 2003. A new bagging technique for apple growing. *South China Fruits* 32: 3, 64.

Johnson, G. R., and B. Johnson. 2000. Sugar maple condition related to deep planting and stem girdling roots. In Johnson, G. R. and R. J. Hauer. 2000. *A Practitioner's Guide to Stem Girdling Roots of Trees*. University of Minnesota Extension Service Publication BU-7501-S.

Johnson, N. C., P. J. Copeland, R. K. Crookston, and F. L. Pfleger. 1992. Mycorrhizae: possible explanation for yield decline with continuous corn and soybean. *Agronomy Journal* 84: 387–390.

Jokinen, R. 1982. Effect of liming on the value of magnesium sulphate and two dolomitic limestones as magnesium sources for ryegrass. *Journal of the Scientific Agricultural Society of Finland* 54: 77–88.

Keever, G. J., G. S. Cobb, J. C. Stephenson, and W. J. Foster. 1989. Effect of hydrophilic polymer amendment on growth of container grown landscape plants. *Journal of Environmental Horticulture* 7: 52–56.

Kenrick, W. 1833. *The New American Orchardist*. Boston: Otis, Broaders.

Khalafalla, M. M., and Hattori, K. 2000. Ethylene inhibitors enhance in vitro root formation on faba bean shoots regenerated on medium containing thidiazuron. *Plant Growth Regulation* 32: 59–63.

Kingman, A. R., and J. Moore. 1982. Isolation, purification, and quantitation of several growth regulator substances in *Ascophyllum nodosum* (Phaeophyta). *Botanica Marina* 25: 149–153.

Kitou, M., and S. Okuno. 1999. Allelopathic potential of phenolic compounds from coffee residue. *Journal of Weed Science and Technology* 44: 349–352.

Kitou, M., and S. Yoshida. 1997. Effect of coffee residue on the growth of several crop species. *Journal of Weed Science and Technology* 42: 25–30.

Kovach, J., C. Petzoldt, J. Degni, and J. Tette. 1992. A method to measure the environmental impact of pesticides. New York's Food and Life Sciences Bulletin 139.

Lawson, W. 1618. *A New Orchard and Garden.* London.

Lee, S. K., R. Tsao, C. Peterson, and J. R. Coats. 1997. Insecticidal activity of monoterpenoids to western corn rootworm (Coleoptera: Chrysomelidae), twospotted spider mite (Acari: Tetranychidae), and house fly (Diptera: Muscidae). *Journal of Economic Entomology* 90: 883–892.

Lemieux, N. C., B. K. Maynard, and W. A. Johnson. 2000. Evaluation of commercial deer repellents on ornamentals in nurseries. *Journal of Environmental Horticulture* 18: 5–8.

Linderman, R. G., and E. A. Davis. 2004. Evaluation of commercial inorganic and organic fertilizer effects on arbuscular mycorrhizae formed by *Glomus intraradices. HortTechnology* 14: 196–202.

Litzow, M., and H. Pellett. 1983. Materials for potential use in sun-scald prevention. *Journal of Arboriculture* 9: 35–38.

Lodeman, E. G., 1906. *The Spraying of Plants.* New York: Macmillan.

Lowery, B., M. Jordan, K. Kelling, and P. Speth. 2004. Use of surfactants to improve water and nitrate use efficiency and decrease leaching. *Proceedings of the Wisconsin Annual Potato Meeting* 17: 123–125.

Lumis, G. P. 1987. Root growth and stimulation at transplanting and effects of wire baskets on tree roots. *Proceedings of the Florida State Horticultural Society* 100: 398.

Lyons, C. G. Jr., R. E. Byers, and K. S. Yoder, 1983. Influence of planting depth on growth and anchorage of young 'Delicious' apple trees. *HortScience* 18: 923–924.

Lyons, C. G. Jr., K. S. Yoder, and R. E. Byers, 1982. Poor anchorage and growth of spur 'Red Delicious' apple trees with deep crown roots. *Scientia Horticulturae,* 18: 45–47.

Ma, J. F., Y. Miyake, and E. Takahashi. 2001. Silicon as a beneficial element for crop plants. In *Silicon in Agriculture*. 2001. Eds. Datnoff, L. E., G. H. Snyder, and G. H. Korndorfer. 17–39. New York: Elsevier.

MacDonald, B. 1986. *Practical Woody Plant Propagation for Nursery Growers*. Portland, OR: Timber Press.

Madanlar, N., Z. Yoldas, E. Durmusoglu, and A. Gul. 2002. Investigations on the natural pesticides against pests in vegetable greenhouses in Izmir (Turkey). *Turkiye Entomoloji Dergisi* 26: 181–195.

Marshall, R. P. 1931. The relation of season of wounding and shellacking to woundwood formation in tree wounds. USDA Technical Bulletin 246.

Massey, L. M. 1925. A cautionary word about fungicides. *The American Rose Annual* 10: 89–92.

McGrath, M. T. 2004. Evaluation of fungicide programs for managing powdery mildew of pumpkin, 2003. *Fungicide and Nematicide Tests* 59: V056.

Edson, D. R. 1917. Starting plants for next springs garden. *House and Garden* 32(August): 42–43.

McIndoo, N. E., and R. C. Roark. 1936. A bibliography of nicotine part II. USDA Bureau of Entomology and Plant Quarantine Circular E-392.

Mengel, K., and E. A. Kirkby. 1987. *Principles of plant nutrition*. Bern, Switzerland: International Potash Institute.

Mercer, P. C. 1979. Attitudes to pruning wounds. *Arboriculture Journal* 3: 457–465.

Metcalf, C. L., and W. P. Flint. 1939. *Destructive and Useful Insects*. New York: McGraw-Hill.

Metcalf, R. L., and R. A. Metcalf. 1993. *Destructive and Useful Insects*. New York: McGraw-Hill.

Mills, H. A., and J. B. Jones. 1996. *Plant Analysis Handbook II*. Athens, GA: Micro Macro International.

Miwa, Y., Y. Kushihashi, and M. Sasagawa. 1992. Behavior of bioelectric potential of the leaf under the sound stimulus. *Environmental Control in Biology* 30: 29–35.

Mmbaga, M. T., and H. Sheng. 2002. Evaluation of biorational products for powdery mildew management in *Cornus florida*. *Journal of Environmental Horticulture* 20: 113–117.

Moore, S. R. 1996. Bicarbonates offer effective disease control. *Grower Talks* (February): 72.

Mozafar, A., and J. J. Oertli. 1993. Thiamin (vitamin B1): translocation and metabolism by soybean seedling. *Journal of Plant Physiology* 142: 438–445.

Nam, M. H., S. K. Jung, S. W. Ra, and H. G. Kim. 2003. Control efficacy of sodium bicarbonate alone and in mixture with polyoxyethylene sorbitan-monolaurate on powdery mildew of strawberry. *Korean Journal of Horticultural Science and Technology* 21: 98–101.

Neilson, J. E. 1928. Paraffin wax: an aid to growth in transplanted trees and shrubs. Northern *Nut Growers Association Proceedings* 19: 44–51.

Nelson, P. V. 2003. *Greenhouse Operation and Management.* Upper Saddle River, NJ: Prentice Hall.

O'Donnell, R. W. 1973. The auxin-like effects of humic preparations from leonardite. *Soil Science* 116: 106–112.

Olkowski, W., S. Daar, and H. Olkowski. 1991. *Common-Sense Pest Control.* Newtown, CT: Taunton Press.

Olsen J. K., J. T. Schaefer, M. N. Hunter, D. G. Edwards, V. J. Galea, and L. M. Muller. 1996. Response of capsicum (*Capsicum annuum* L.), sweet corn (*Zea mays* L.), and tomato (*Lycopersicon esculentum* Mill.) to inoculation with vesicular-arbuscular mycorrhizae. *Australian Journal of Agricultural Research* 47: 651–671.

Owen, N. P., C. S. Sadof, and M. J. Raupp. 1991. The effect of plastic tree wrap on borer incidence in dogwood. *Journal of Arboriculture* 17: 29–31.

Paine, T. D., C. C. Hanlon, D. R. Pittenger, D. M. Ferrin, and M. K. Malinowski. 1992. Consequences of water and nitrogen management on growth and aesthetic quality of drought-tolerant woody landscape plants. *Journal of Environmental Horticulture* 10: 94–99.

Parkinson, J. 1629. *Paradisi in sole Paradisus Terrestris.* London: Humfrey Lownes and Robert Young.

Pasini, C., F. D'Aquila, P. Curir, and M. L. Gullino. 1997. Effectiveness of antifungal compounds against rose powdery mildew (*Sphaerotheca pannosa* var. *rosae*) in glasshouses. *Crop Protection* 16: 251–256.

Peets, E. 1925. *Practical Tree Repair.* New York: McBride.

Percival, G. C., and G. A. Fraser. 2005. Use of sugars to improve root growth and increase transplant success of birch. *Journal of Arboriculture* 31: 66-77.

Perry, K. B., A. R. Bonanno, and D. W. Monks. 1992. Two putative cryoprotectants do not provide frost and freeze protection in tomato and pepper. *HortScience* 27: 26–27.

Peterson, J., R. Belz, F. Walker, and K. Hurle. 2001. Weed suppression by release of isothiocyanates from turnip-rape mulch. *Agronomy Journal* 93: 37–43.

Pharand, B., O. Carisse, and N. Benhamou. 2002. Cytological aspects of compost-mediated induced resistance against Fusarium crown and root rot in tomato. *Phytopathology* 92: 424–438.

Ponder, H. G., C. H. Gilliam, and H. J. Davies. 1983. Factors affecting postharvest stress of summer dug *Photinia*. *HortScience* 18: 83–85.

Quintinye, J. 1690. *Instruction pour les Jardins Fruitiers et Potagers*. Paris.

Rankin, M. A., and S. Rankin. 1980. Some factors affecting presumed migratory flight activity of the convergent ladybeetle *Hippodamia convergens*. Biological Bulletin 158: 356–369.

Raven, P. H., R. F. Evert, and S. E. Eichorn. 1986. *Biology of Plants*. New York: Worth.

Relf, D., and B. Appleton. 2001. Managing winter injury to trees and shrubs. *Virginia Cooperative Extension Environmental Horticulture* 426-500.

Retallack, D. 1973. *The Sound of Music and Plants*. Marina del Rey, CA: DeVross.

Reyes-Hernandez, A., A. B. Manes-Suarez, M. Gessa-Galvez, P. Cairo-Cairo, J. Machado-de-Armas, R. Quinones-Ramos, and J. Machado-de-Armas. 2002. Effects of the application of solid coffee residues as a source of organic matter. *Centro Agricola* 29: 92–93.

Ries, S., R. Baughan, M. G. Nair, and R. Schutzki. 2001. Repelling animals from crops using plant extracts. *HortTechnology* 11: 302–307.

Rosa, E. A. S., and P. M. F. Rodrigues. 1999. Towards a more sustainable agriculture system: the effect of glucosinolates on the control of soil-borne diseases. *Journal of Horticultural Science and Biotechnology* 74: 667–674.

Rovesti, L., T. Fiorini, G. Bettini, E. W. Heinzpeter, and F. Tagliente. 1990. Compatibility of *Steinernema* spp. and *Heterorhabditis* spp. with pesticides. *Informatore Fitopatologico* 40(9): 55–61.

Ruffin, E. 1832. *An Essay on Calcareous Manures*. Reprint. Cambridge, MA: Belknap Press, 1961.

Russel, G. E. 1978. Some effects of applied potassium and sodium chloride on yellow rust in winter wheat. *Annuls of Applied Biology* 90: 163–168.

Saftner, R. A., and R. E. Wyse. 1984. Effect of plant hormones on sucrose uptake by sugar beet root tissue discs. *Plant Physiology* 74: 951–955.

Sanderson, K. J., and P. E. Jameson. 1986. The cytokinins in a liquid seaweed extract: could they be the active ingredients? *Acta-Horticulturae* 179: 113–116

Sanderson, K. J., P. E. Jameson, and J. A. Zabkiewicz. 1987. Auxin in a seaweed extract: identification and quantitation of indole-3-acetic acid by gas chromatography/mass spectrometry. *Journal of Plant Physiology* 129: 363–367.

Scagel, C. F., and R. G. Linderman. 2001. Modification of root IAA concentrations, tree growth, and survival by application of plant growth regulating substances to container-grown conifers. *New Forests* 21: 159–186.

Scagel, C. F., R. G. Linderman, and R. K. Scagel. 2000. Ten-year growth and survival of Douglas-fir seedlings treated with plant growth regulating substances at transplant. *Canadian Journal of Forest Research* 30: 1778–1787.

Sclar, D. C., D. Gerace, A. Tupy, K. Wilson, S. A. Spriggs, R. J. Bishop, and W. S. Cranshaw. 1999. Effects of application of various reduced-risk pesticides to tomato, with notes on control of greenhouse whitefly. *Hort-Technology* 9: 185–189.

Shapiro Ilan D. I., R. F. Mizell, T. E. Cottrell, and D. L. Horton. 2004. Measuring field efficacy of *Steinernema feltiae* and *Steinernema riobrave* for suppression of plum curculio, *Conotrachelus nenuphar*, larvae. *Biological Control* 30: 496–503.

Sharma, A. R., and R. N Trigiano. 1999. Rooting flowering dogwood (Cornus florida) microshoots. *Proceedings SNA Research Conference* 44: 376–377.

Shigo, A. L. 1981. To paint or not to paint tree wounds, pruning cuts. *Brooklyn Botanic Garden Record* 37(2): 20–22.

Spurway, C. H. 1944. Soil reaction (pH) preferences of plants. Michigan State College Agricultural Experiment Station. Technical Bulletin 306.

Steinhaus, E. A. 1949. *Principles of Insect Pathology*. New York: McGraw-Hill.

Stephens, J. M. 1994. Organic vegetable gardening. Florida Cooperative Extension Service. University of Florida Institute of Food and Agricultural Sciences Circular 375.

Struve, D. K., and R. T. Joly. 1992. Transplanted red oak seedlings mediate transplant shock by reducing leaf surface area and altering carbon allocation. *Canadian Journal of Forest Research* 22: 1441–1448.

Struve D. K., R. D. Kelly, and B. C. Moser. 1983. Promotion of root regeneration in difficult-to-transplant species. *Combined Proceedings of the International Plant Propagators' Society* 33: 433–439.

Swanson, B. T., C. Rosen, R Munter, and C. Lane. 1986. Soil testing and fertilizer applications for nursery management and production. University of Minnesota Agricultural Extension Service Bulletin AG-BU-2830.

Swihart, R. K., and M. R. Conover. 1990. Reducing deer damage to yews and apple trees: testing Big Game Deer Repellent, Ro-pel and soap as repellents. Wildlife Society Bulletin 18: 156–162.

Thimann, K. V., and J. B. Koepfli. 1935. Identity of the growth-promoting and root-forming substances of plants. *Nature* 135: 101–102.

Tompkins, P., and C. Bird. 1973. *The Secret Life of Plants*. New York: Perennial.

Tripepi R. R., M. W. George, R. K. Dumroese, and D. L. Wenny. 1991. Birch seedling response to irrigation frequency and a hydrophilic polymer amendment in a container medium. *Journal of Environmental Horticulture* 9: 119–123.

Tuskan, G. A., and P. L. Ellis. 1991. Auxin-impregnated hygroscopic gel: effects on ponderosa pine and common hackberry seedlings. *New Forests* 5: 359–367.

United Kingdom. 1985. Food and Environmental Protection Act 1985. London: HMSO.

Uniyal, S. P., and A. C. Mishra. 2003. Response of potato to soil moisture and temperature as affected by different mulches. *Journal of the Indian Potato Association* 30: 315–318.

Unruh, J. B., Christians, N. E., and H. T. Horner. 1997. Herbicidal effects of the dipeptide alaninyl-alanine on perennial ryegrass seedlings. *Crop Science* 37: 208–212.

van Iersel, M. 1998a. Plant growth stimulator effects on post-transplant growth and flowering of petunia and impatiens plugs. *HortTechnology* 8: 45–47.

———. 1998b. Antitranspirants do not reduce transplant shock of impatiens seedlings in a greenhouse. *HortTechnology* 8: 570–573.

Voss, M. C., H. H. Hoppe, and B. Ulber. 1998. Estimation of slug activity and slug abundance. *Zeitschrift fur Pflanzenkrankheiten und Pflanzenschutz* 105: 314–321.

Wakasawa, H., K. Takahashi, and K. Mochizuki. 1998. Application and composting conditions of coffee grounds 1. Application of coffee grounds in soil. *Japanese Journal of Soil Science and Plant Nutrition* 69: 1–6.

Walker, E. 1905. Asparagus and salt. Arkansas Agricultural Experiment Station Bulletin 86: 31–36.

Walker, R. L., and E. A. Powell. 2001. Soil water retention on gold mine surfaces in the Mojave Desert. *Restoration Ecology* 9: 95–103.

Wallis, M. G., D. J. Horne, and K. W. McAuliffe. 1990. A study of water repellency and its amelioration in a yellow-brown sand. 2. Use of wetting agents and their interaction with some aspects of irrigation. *New Zealand Journal of Agricultural Science* 33: 145–150.

Wang, S. J. 2003. Preliminary experiment of bagging culture for kiwifruit. *South China Fruits* 32: 2, 47.

Wang, Y. T. 1989. Medium and hydrogel affect production and wilting of tropical ornamental plants. *HortScience* 24: 941–944.

Wang, Y., R. Gaugler, and L. W. Cui. 1994. Variations in immune response of

Popillia japonica and *Acheta domesticus* to *Heterorhabditis bacteriophora* and *Steinernema* species. *Journal of Nematology* 26: 11–18.

Ware, G. W. 2000. *The Pesticide Book*. Fresno, CA: Thomson Publications.

Weed, C. M. 1915. *Insects and Insecticides*. New York: Orange Judd.

Weryszko-Chmielewska, E. 1990. The effects of some frequencies of audible continuous sound on the growth of seedling of wheat. *Acta Agrobotanica* 43: 37–51.

Westwood, M. N. 1993. *Temperate Zone Pomology*. Portland, OR: Timber Press.

Widmer, T. L., J. H. Graham, and D. J. Mitchell. 1998. Composted municipal waste reduces infection of citrus seedlings by *Phytophthora nicotianae*. *Plant disease* 82: 683–688.

Wilen, C. A., U. K. Schuch, and C. L. Elmore. 1999. Mulches and subirrigation control weeds in container production. *Journal of Environmental Horticulture* 17: 174–180.

William, H. T. 1871a. Iron for pear trees. *The Horticulturist* 26: 186.

———. 1871b. Mulch as manure. *The Horticulturist* 26: 186.

Wilson, L. T., P. J. Trichilo, and D. Gonzalez. 1991. Natural enemies of spider mites on cotton: density regulation or causal association. *Environmental Entomology* 20: 849–856.

Wright, A. N., A. X. Niemiera, J. R. Harris, and R. D. Wright. 1999. Micronutrient fertilization of woody seedlings essential regardless of pine bark pH. *Journal of Environmental Horticulture* 17: 69–72.

Wyrzykowska, B., K. Szymczyk, H. Ichichashi, J. Falandysz, B. Skwarzec, and S. Yamasaki. 2001. Application of ICP sector field MS and principal component analysis for studying interdependences among 23 trace elements in Polish beers. *Journal of Agricultural and Food Chemistry* 49: 3425–3431.

Xin, H. M., and X. H. Zhang. 2003. Experiment of bagging culture of Meirenzhi grape variety. *China Fruits* 4: 26–27.

Yunta, F., M. A. Sierra, M. Gomez-Gallego, R. Alcazar, S. Garcia-Marco, and J. J. Lucena. 2003. Methodology to screen new iron chelates: prediction of their behavior in nutrient solution and soil conditions. *Journal of Plant Nutrition* 26: 1955–1968.

Zhang, D., R. E. Moran, and L. B. Stack. 2004. Effect of phosphorus fertilization on growth and flowering of Scaevola aemula R. Br. 'New Wonder'. *HortScience* 39: 1728–1731.

Zhang, X., E. H. Ervin, and R. E. Schmidt. 2003a. Physiological effects of liquid applications of a seaweed extract and a humic acid on creeping bentgrass. *Journal of the American Society for Horticultural Science* 128: 492–496.

————. 2003b. Plant growth regulators can enhance the recovery of Kentucky bluegrass sod from heat injury. *Crop Science* 43: 952–956.

Zilliox, L. 2000. Bag apples for spray-free apple maggot control. University of Minnesota Extension Service Yard and Garden Line News 2(1): 1.

Ziv, O., and A. Hagiladi. 1993. Controlling powdery mildew in euonymus with polymer coatings and bicarbonate solutions. *HortScience* 28: 124–126.

Ziv, O., and T. A. Zitter. 1992. Effects of bicarbonates and film-forming polymers on cucurbit foliar diseases. *Plant Disease* 26: 513–517.

Index